INTERNATIONAL HEALTH PERSPECTIVES: *Vol. 1*
An Introduction in Five Volumes

1

WORLDWIDE OVERVIEW
OF HEALTH AND DISEASE

AUTHORS

STEPHEN C. JOSEPH, M.D., M.P.H. (Office of International Health Programs, Harvard School of Public Health)

A pediatrician, Dr. Joseph's international experience began with the Peace Corps in Nepal, continued with appointment on the medical faculty in Yaounde, Cameroon (1970-73) and subsequently assumed a diversified and active character through projects at his present institution.

DIETER KOCH-WESER, M.D., Ph.D. (Department of Preventive and Social Medicine, Harvard Medical School)

Dr. Koch-Weser received his early training and clinical experience in Brazil. He has significant international experience including service with the Brazilian government, the World Health Organization, various United States agencies and a large international medical program at his institution.

NED WALLACE, M.D., M.P.H. (University of Wisconsin School of Medicine, Office of International Health)

Dr. Wallace has eight years of international experience as a practitioner and administrator of a rural hospital in eastern Nicaragua (with emphasis on general medicine and surgery). He has drawn on this experience to add depth to discussions of health in the affluent vs developing countries.

ASSOCIATION OF AMERICAN MEDICAL COLLEGES

INTERNATIONAL HEALTH PERSPECTIVES:
An Introduction in Five Volumes

Wendy H. Waddell, Robert G. Pierleoni and Emanuel Suter, Editors

A SELF-INSTRUCTIONAL COURSE

1

WORLDWIDE OVERVIEW OF HEALTH AND DISEASE

Stephen C. Joseph, M.D., M.P.H.

Dieter Koch-Weser, M.D., Ph.D.

Ned Wallace, M.D., M.P.H.

 SPRINGER PUBLISHING COMPANY/ New York

173150

Development of this international health course was made
possible through the support of the Fogarty International
Center. The information contained in this publication in no
way reflects the views of the Fogarty International Center,
The National Institutes of Health, The Department of Health,
Education and Welfare, or any other Federal agency.

This is a revised edition of <u>An Introduction to International
Health: Principles of a Cross-Cultural and Comparative Approach
to Health Problems</u> by the Association of American Medical
Colleges, printed from camera-ready copy prepared for the
publisher by AAMC.

Springer Publishing Company, Inc.
200 Park Avenue South
New York, New York 10003

Library of Congress Catalog Card Number: 77-85143

International Standard Book Numbers: 0-8261-2491-7 (volume 1)
0-8261-2490-9 (5-volume se

Printed in the United States of America

PREFACE

The Fogarty International Center for Advanced Study
in the Health Sciences was established as a memorial to
the late Congressman John E. Fogarty of Rhode Island. It
had been Mr. Fogarty's desire to create within the National
Institutes of Health a center for research in biology and
medicine dedicated to international cooperation and colla-
oration in the interest of the health of mankind.

As an institution for advanced study, the Fogarty
International Center has embraced the major themes of biomedical research, medical education, environmental health,
societal factors influencing health and disease, geographic
health problems, international health research and education, and preventive medicine. The Center has published
proceedings of conferences and seminars devoted to these
subjects.

The Fogarty Center endorses the objectives of this
interdisciplinary, self-instructional syllabus and is
pleased to have provided support for its development.

Milo D. Leavitt, Jr., M.D.
Director
Fogarty International Center
National Institutes of Health

EDITORS

WENDY H. WADDELL (AAMC Staff, Division of Educational
  Resources and Programs)

Ms. Waddell previously administered the AAMC international
student fellowship program (1972-1974) and developed
country-specific materials for the fellows to use prior
to going overseas.

ROBERT G. PIERLEONI, Ed.D. (University of Kansas Office of
  Health Sciences Education)

Dr. Pierleoni provides academic consulting to faculty
on the development of instructional materials, the
measurement and evaluation of student progress and the
assessment of teaching effectiveness. He also designs
and conducts faculty development programs and educational
research studies.

EMANUEL SUTER, M.D. (AAMC Staff, Director, Division of
  Educational Resources and Programs)

Dr. Suter directed the AAMC Division of International
Medical Education during the development of the course
and has carried overall responsibility for its coordination, development, testing and revision.

FOREWORD

nearly a century, progress in medicine and medical care
been spearheaded by scientific advances in the biomedical
ences. The beginning of this era is arbitrarily recognized
h the discoveries of Koch, Pasteur and others--first in
ectious diseases and physiology, and later, in biochemistry.
culmination of these advances has been the elucidation of
helical structure for DNA and the recognition of a univer-
ity among elemental biological mechanisms.

ay, major new thrusts in health care are coming from socio-
tural, economic and political forces. Every country,
ther old or new, developed or developing, rich or poor,
confronting problems surrounding the provision of medical
ences to its people. Serious difficulties are being met
making health care a right for all people and not a pro-
e. Escalation of medical care costs around the world
ws more heavily on every nation's resources. The aging
the world population places a heavier burden on the rela-
ely fewer people in their productive years to meet the
ts of medical care for the aged.

re appears to be no powerful new calculus waiting to be
lied to solve these problems. The equations of the health
nomists will not provide answers to essentially moral
stions that center around the difficult issue of how much
our wealth we will or can spend to relieve human suffering
preserve human life.

commonality of the problems makes it essential that all
ions work together in seeking solutions. No country has
unquestioned preeminence in the field; ideas and solutions
come from any quarter.

Rapid changes in the health care dynamics of this country and abroad make it desirable for students of medicine to be introduced to issues of health and health care on a worldwide basis. For this reason, the Association has worked with international health faculty throughout the U.S. in producing a course that places U.S. health care against a cross-cultural backdrop of health systems and economic priorities around the world.

The authors and producers of this self-instructional course have employed an ecologic approach to health and disease issues which should help to prepare students both for experience abroad and for health service at home. We in the AAMC are hopeful that these self-instructional materials will prove themselves to be a helpful addition to the educational tools presently available in understanding the health problems that confront us in the United States.

June 1977

JOHN A. D. COOPER, M.D.
PRESIDENT
ASSOCIATION OF AMERICAN
MEDICAL COLLEGES

TABLE OF CONTENTS

.e international health course consists of five volumes,
.ch containing independent but related units of content.
.roughout the course, the terms "category/volume" are used
.terchangeably, as are the terms "unit/chapter."

ix

IT I/5.   INTERNATIONAL COOPERATION IN HEALTH

INTRODUCTION

e international health course is expected to serve two
ictions:

To provide introductory materials for students planning
observe or participate in the health care system of
ither country, or intending to pursue a career in inter-
tional health, and

To provide supporting material for some of the community
alth courses which are being planned or have already been
plemented by a number of institutions. (The second title
the course, "Principles of a Cross-Cultural and Comparative
proach to Health Problems," implies that many of the
rinciples" are presented in an international context, but
e equally pertinent to the immediate health concerns of
e United States.

e course is designed to stimulate self-learning and to
courage periodic reflection on health problems and con-
pts through interspersed questioning. Because this self-
structional format makes tutorial guidance by an instructor
rticularly effective, the course can be used either as a
eestanding exercise or in conjunction with other course
terials. For faculty who wish to use the course formally
thin the curriculum, an evaluation packet can be obtained
writing to the Division of Educational Resources and
ograms, Association of American Medical Colleges, One
pont Circle, N.W., Suite 200, Washington, D. C. 20036.

e need for an international health course gradually became
parent to AAMC over a several year period during which the
sociation sponsored international fellowships for third
d fourth year U.S. medical students in other countries.
ten, it was learned, U.S. students had difficulty in com-
ring health information from other countries with our U.S.
tuation. Repeatedly, these students pointed to the need
r better preparation prior to overseas travel.

Following indepth discussions by the Midwest Universities Consortium on International Activities as to the scope and content of such a course, and after more comprehensive discussions with international health faculty at the AAMC Annual Meetings of 1972 and 1973, support for the development of the course was obtained from the Fogarty International Center, National Institutes of Health in May 1975. The course underwent a pilot test phase in early 1977 during which more than 140 students from 15 medical and public health schools used the materials and generated suggestions for this revised first edition.

The development of this international health course was made possible through the efforts of many people over a two year period. In addition to the contributions of our international health experts, we want to thank Dr. Donald Pitcairn of the Fogarty International Center for his continuing support and encouragement. We are grateful to the faculty members and students at fifteen institutions around the country, who agreed to take the course and provide us with constructive criticism for its revision. Dr. James DeNio and Ms. Carol Payne of the University of Kansas Medical Center helped us with the evaluation materials and Ms. Mary Staples of the AAMC provided able and cooperative assistance with all of the administrative details of the project. We also must acknowledge the patience and perseverance of Ms. Veda Tripp in typing the manuscript and Ms. Lesley Knox in tabulating the pilot test results and producing the final typed copy for these volumes.

WENDY H. WADDELL
Association of American Medical Colleges

ROBERT G. PIERLEONI, Ed.D.
University of Kansas Medical Center

EMANUEL SUTER, M.D.
Association of American Medical Colleges

June 1977

UNIT I/1. HEALTH PROBLEMS OF THE RICH AND POOR COUNTRIES

BY

STEPHEN C. JOSEPH, M.D., M.P.H.
DIETER KOCH-WESER, M.D., PH.D.
NED WALLACE, M.D., M.P.H.

CONTENTS

OBJECTIVES

Throughout the world there are dramatic differences in the health status and health problems of different populations. Category 1 is intended to provide a general overview of these different health patterns, and this introductory unit is aimed more specifically at distinguishing between the major health problems of the rich and poor countries. This material will provide the necessary background for succeeding units in this and other categories.

As a result of working with this unit, you should be able to provide at least a preliminary answer to each of the following questions:

1. Characteristics of the rich and poor countries: can we define "development?"

2. Can we define "health?"

3. What factors influence health?

4. How can we measure and compare these factors?

5. What are the major world patterns of morbidity and mortality?

6. What resources do countries have available to deal with health problems?

As you read, try to identify the major health and development characteristics as they vary between rich and poor countries. You will be asked to draw on this knowledge for an examination of health problems discussed in their international perspective.

CHARACTERISTICS OF RICH AND POOR COUNTRIES

eparatory to a global overview of health and disease, one
st attempt to define terms and boundaries. The map below
picts a rough grouping of the world's nations into "poor"
d "affluent" countries. Make a mental note of the pat-
rns this map indicates.

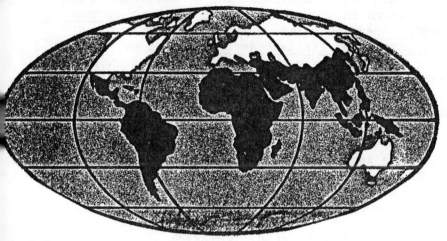

Approximate location of poor countries.

Affluent countries.

e developing poor countries largely fall in the tropical
eas of the world - in Africa, Asia, and Latin America be-
een the Tropics of Cancer and Capricorn - while the af-
uent nations are to be found in North America, Europe
ncluding Russia) and countries such as Japan, Australia,
w Zealand, Israel and the Republic of South Africa. While
ny of the developing countries exhibit a modest level of
dustrialization, a major portion of their population is

involved in traditional subsistence agriculture. In contrast, most of the affluent nations are highly technological industrial states and often have a significant mechanization of agriculture.

Because of the close relationship between economic and health factors, a discussion of the health problems of individual communities and nations would be meaningless if not characterized within the framework of the economically "rich and poor." Terms in widespread use are <u>developing countries</u> or <u>developing areas</u> to refer to "poor" populations and <u>affluent countries</u> or <u>affluent areas</u> to refer to "rich."* However, no single term is universally accepted and, of course, there are political and social connotations to such classifications which make them objectionable to some individuals and groups.

What distinguishes a country as being rich or poor? Unfortunately, there is no absolute agreement concerning the criteria which classify an individual, community, or country as being either rich or poor. However, some rough descriptions can be used for purposes of comparison.

ECONOMIC CHARACTERISTICS

The most widely used measures to distinguish affluent from developing countries are economic. Most frequently applied on a national basis is the per capita Gross National Product (per capita GNP), the value of the goods and services produced annually by a country, divided by the population. In

---

* The term "developed" countries is often used to refer to the affluent countries; we prefer to avoid this term as it implies a static achievement which is not at all the case.

absence of a more satisfactory indicator, the per capita
is useful, though its accuracy is often hampered by in-
urate data, shifting international exchange rates, and
pecially in countries where much of the population lives
ubsistence agricultural life) difficulty in estimating or
luating "non-cash" factors. Since all countries have a
ll, wealthy segment of the population, the per capita GNP
not be considered a reflection of average individual in-
e of most of the country.

n when "rich and poor" is defined in purely economic
ms, however, the validity of the economic indicator is
inished by the marked differences within a country, be-
en regions, communities, population groups and individuals.
tainly some countries are predominantly rich and others
dominantly poor, but there are underprivileged population
ups everywhere. Table 1 below illustrates that this is
e in developing as in affluent countries.

TABLE 1

PERCENT SHARE OF NATIONAL INCOME DISTRIBUTED AMONG:

	PER CAPITA GNP ($U.S.)	LOWEST 40% OF POPULATION	MIDDLE 40% OF POPULATION
ilippines (1971)	239	11.6	34.6
bon (1968)	497	8.8	23.7
nezuela (1970)	1,004	7.9	27.1
nzania (1967)	89	13.0	26.0
minican Republic (1969)	323	12.2	30.3
gentina (1970)	1,079	16.5	36.1
ailand (1970)	180	17.0	37.5
goslavia (1967)	529	18.5	40.0
A (1970)	4,850	19.7	41.5

Source: M.S. Ahluwalia, in Redistribution with Growth,
edited by H. Chenery et al. Oxford University Press
London, 1974. Reprinted with permission.

Abandonment of the rural areas by uncontrolled migration to the cities, and general neglect of the same rural areas in most developing countries has expanded the economic diversity and inequality within those countries, creating both accentuated rural poverty and mushrooming urban poverty with consequent increases in health problems.

An objection to purely economic measures of "development" is raised by those who feel that increased economic productivity is usually achieved by further deterioration of the environment, and that true development is directed toward man living in equilibrium with his environment. Unfortunately, overall indices which indicate environmental equality or environmental equilibrium do not exist. Nevertheless, an increasing number of individuals and countries are taking into account improvements in such areas as education, health, science, the arts, infrastructure in the private and governmental sectors, and other social aspects of life in an attempt to reflect more nearly "development."

Table 2 on the opposite page presents data for several social indicators according to national wealth. Compare the figures for the United States and Bangladesh. Consider the magnitude of the difference between them in per capita income.

1. How do the figures for per capita GNP compare with literacy rates for the two countries?

2. What pattern do you notice in terms of:

   (a) birth rates?
   (b) death rates?

After you have jotted down your answers, see p. 8.

TABLE 2

ECONOMIC AND SOCIAL INDICATORS
SELECTED COUNTRIES, 1970-75 (VARIOUS YEARS)

(...OR COUNTRIES)	ANNUAL PER CAPITA GNP ($U.S.)	LITERACY (% POPULATION)	ANNUAL BIRTHS PER 1000 POPULATION	ANNUAL DEATHS PER 1000 POPULATION	INFANT MORTALITY RATE[*]
...ANGLADESH	70	22	50	28	132
...PPER VOLTA	70	20	49	26	160
...GANISTAN	80	8	49	24	182
...THIOPIA	80	5	49	26	181
...EPAL	80	9	43	20	187
...AIRE	100	40	45	21	160
...DIA	110	28	40	16	139
...ITI	130	10	36	17	150
...AKISTAN	130	5	47	17	200
...INA (P.R.C)	170	84	27	10	55
...NYA	170	25	49	16	135
...OLIVIA	200	91	44	18	31
...HILIPPINES	220	72	44	11	78
...HAILAND	220	68	43	11	65
...OROCCO	270	14	46	16	149
...RKEY	370	46	39	13	119
...OLOMBIA	400	73	41	9	76
...ATEMALA	420	38	43	14	79
...AZIL	530	32	37	9	108
...XICO	750	78	42	9	61
(...LY RICH COUNTRIES)[#]					
...GERIA	130	25	50	23	180
...AN	490	23	45	16	139
...UDI ARABIA	550	15	50	20	152
...NEZUELA	1,240	76	36	7	50
...BYAN ARAB REP.	1,830	27	45	15	130
...WAIT	4,090	47	47	5	44
(...LUENT COUNTRIES)					
...GOSLAVIA	810	80	18	9	43
...SR	1,530	99	18	8	26
...ECHOSLOVAKIA	2,180	100	17	11	21
...PAN	2,320	93	19	7	12
...ITED KINGDOM	2,600	99	16	12	18
...THERLANDS	2,840	98	17	9	12
...STRALIA	2,980	93	21	8	17
...ANCE	3,620	97	17	11	16
...EDEN	4,480	99	14	11	10
...S.A.	5,590	98	16	9	18

* Deaths under 1 year of age/1000 live births
# The per capita GNP figures for 1972 do not reflect the quintupling oil prices in 1973-74

Source: Modified from The U.S. & World Development: Agenda for Action, 1975 Overseas Development Council, pp. 198-207.

1. *You should have indicated that the differences in per capita GNP are directly (as opposed to inversely) related to the differences in literacy rates.*

2. *(a) the birth rate is inversely related to the per capita GNP.*
   (b) The death rate is inversely related to the per capita GNP.

Note that in general those countries with the highest GNP also have higher literacy, lower population growth and lower death rates, while the opposite is true for low income countries.

POPULATION CHARACTERISTICS

In the developing countries, a high proportion of the population remains rural. However, the urbanization trends of affluent countries are now also present in most of the developing countries. Traditional village society persists in many poorer regions, with accompanying social patterns such as the extended family system. In contrast, the extended family organizational pattern of most affluent nations has diminished considerably since the turn of the century.

A characterization of rich and poor countries has been further complicated in very recent years in that in a group of countries "the newly rich " present a combination of characteristics of the affluent and developing groups. These countries - best represented by the OPEC (Organization of Petroleum Exporting Countries) nations - have recently acquired great wealth and yet lag in technological and other parameters of development. They still retain to a greater or lesser extent the life style and overall pattern of poverty and (relatively) rudimentary technologic infrastructure to be found in the developing countries which lack these economic resources.

WORKING EXERCISE

fore proceeding further, please take a few moments to
view the general characteristics of rich and poor
untries just discussed above and summarize your present
derstanding of these factors by completing Table 3 on
e next page. (This is intended as a working exercise,
we suggest you tear out the table and keep it handy in
se you want to add to or change your descriptions as
u proceed through the unit.) Later, you will be asked
review and compare your table with our unit synopsis.

TABLE 3

CHARACTERISTICS OF THE AFFLUENT AND POOR COUNTRIES

AFFLUENT COUNTRIES	POOR COUNTRIES
ECONOMIC CHARACTERISTICS	
POPULATION CHARACTERISTICS	
HEALTH/DISEASE PATTERNS	

WHAT IS HEALTH?

atever efforts are made to investigate or define the con-
pt of "quality of life," the health of the population is
nsistently a key factor. In considering the World Health
ganization's definition that *"health is a state of optimal
ysical, mental and social well-being, and not merely the
sence of disease or infirmity,"* it is clear that health
synonomous with "quality of life." Quite acceptable in
philosophical sense, this definition, however, is difficult
employ in a practical sense, especially if one wishes to
tablish objectives or checkpoints for measuring health
atus or changes in the health status of populations.

the other hand, the definition is constructive in that
emphasizes that the health of individuals and communities
pends on the interaction of many biological and non-bio-
gical factors. Health professionals learn a great deal
out the biological factors (down to the molecular level),
t many often remain ignorant of the non-biological factors
ich influence health - that is, the social, political,
onomic, educational, cultural and religious factors.

FACTORS INFLUENCING HEALTH

e global problems of contaminated water and sewage systems,
lnutrition, overpopulation, poor housing, and the major
alth problems of affluent countries that are intimately
lated to life style (e.g. accidents, alcohol, tobacco,
ug abuse, and toxic effects of environmental pollution)
e proof that non-biological as well as biological factors
ve a critical impact upon the health of individuals and
mmunities. The following environmental factors, all

closely dependent on economic conditions, interact in a
significant way with health.*

WATER SUPPLY

In developing countries where large segments of the population are rural and isolated, the difficulty and costs of
providing potable water are high, since separate water
sources are often required for small numbers of people.
Those living at a subsistence level can scarcely afford the
luxury of a well or of piped water; the provision and
maintenance of water systems for villages and towns by
local, state or national government is usually much too
expensive to consider. In many countries where efforts
have been made to improve water supplies, partial or
complete failures of some projects and high costs have
deterred a high priority emphasis on water. An inadequate
supply of safe water impedes adequate cleaning of food,
cooking utensils, and hands. In addition, it increases
the risk of enteric infection. Significant decreases in
morbidity and mortality from enteric infection have been
observed consistently in populations when adequate and
safe water supplies become available.

WASTE DISPOSAL

Inadequate waste disposal, primarily of excreta, influences
health by facilitating fecally spread diseases. Parasitic
infestation by hookworm and roundworm require man in their
life cycles. Pathogenic bacteria from human and animal
feces can pollute sources of drinking water. These elem-
entary observations have provided the foundation for the

---

*   These factors are considered more fully in Category III,
    "Ecologic Determinants of Health Problems" and Category IV,
    "Sociocultural Influences on Health and Health Care"

nitation systems in the industrialized world, which are
w developed to the extent that major health problems caused
inadequate waste disposal are greatly diminished. However,
thin the poor countries, where financial resources of
lividuals and governments are insufficient, the morbidity
1 mortality and the threat of epidemics remain high and
ll continue to be so. It is probable that improvement in
e quality of water supply and waste disposal would influence
a greater degree the health of more people in the devel-
ing world than all actions of members of the health prof-
sions. This observation carries important implications
r planning in poor countries where resources for health
rvices are severely limited. The historical observation
1 analysis of the response of disease patterns to such
anges as improvements in water supply and sanitation can
ovide valuable guidelines for policy and planning decisions
countries with limited resources.

TRITION

lnutrition as a health problem involves not only bio-
emical and metabolic disturbances, but also economic pro-
ems in food production, distribution, and consumption.
ltural and religious influences on food preferences and
jections, food distribution within the family, the lack of
derstanding of nutritional values, and even the unfortunate
ndency to use food as a political weapon are other factors
sociated with nutritional deficiency. In addition to the
vious protein-energy (sometimes called protein-calorie)
tritional diseases of kwashiorkor and marasmus, under-
trition and malnutrition influence health primarily by
creasing the normal body responses to infection.

ause many types of food are seasonal and often difficult
store, a constant year-round supply of food is expensive
maintain. High costs of production, storage and trans-
rtation of food force a reliance on local, cheap and often

inadequate food. In urban areas overpopulated by migration to the cities, production of food is not possible, so that all food must be purchased. Floods, droughts, storms, and storage losses can reduce available food and increase its cost to a prohibitive level.

Adequate nutrition requires a balanced mix of foods which often cannot be secured by those with limited incomes. As costs of production, transportation and storage rise, the impact of poverty on nutrition and subsequently on health will also rise.

POPULATION

The entire issue of overpopulation probably is more a religious, political, social, cultural and economic problem than a medical one and its resolution will depend more on consideration of these factors than on health measures. The exponential growth of populations during the past decades in the poor countries and earlier in industrialized nations of the world, has been determined mainly by falling death rates, and these in turn have been influenced more by improved nutritional and living standards than by medical measures. The population "explosion" places a great - perhaps unbearable - strain upon nutritional and economic resources. However, if this population pressure can be checked by programs of family planning and by more equitable distribution and efficient use of global resources, there may be some cause for optimism. It has become a consistent observation that family size decreases as affluence increases. In fact, this phenomenon has stimulated some economists and others to gear family planning programs toward increasing the economic level of a community or country. Large families are vital to subsistence in poor agrarian countries because they provide an inexpensive labor pool. As parents grow older and are less able to provide for their own subsistence,

pport by their children becomes more and more important -
pecially in those countries where government programs of
d age security are non-existent or modest - the more
ildren, the greater the support.

situations of high infant and childhood mortality,
milies are aware that more pregnancies are required to
sure children who will live to productive adulthood,
ereby continuing a high birth rate.

USING AND LIFE STYLE

owded and poorly ventilated housing provides a breeding
ound for vectors of many diseases and promotes the direct
ansmission of other diseases. Because adequate housing
rrelates closely with income, the poor often cannot
tain it.

entirely new pattern of predominant diseases and causes
death has arisen from the complex changes in individual
d societal life styles accompanying industrialization,
banization, and technological "modernization." As the
uses of these diseases are multifactorial in nature, so
so their possible solutions involve economic, political
d socio-cultural factors that go far beyond "medicine"
the traditional sense.

ASSESSMENT OF HEALTH*

be able to effectively act on the health factors noted
ove, one must first be in a position to obtain a reason-
ly accurate assessment of health. While it may be

For a further discussion of health assessment, consult
the units in Category II, "Assessment of Health Status
and Needs."

possible to assess the health status of an individual,
it is far more difficult to provide measures for a group
of people - a family, a community, or an entire nation.
Without a common standard of health, attempts to
determine, measure or compare it are not very meaningful.
Nevertheless, information obtained from existing assessment
indices is needed for many purposes.

HEALTH PLANNING -- to assist in the decision-making
process of where and how health
resources should be directed.

HEALTH PROGRAM EVALUATION -- to determine the influence
of a health program on the
health status of at least
some members of a community.

MONITORING OF HEALTH CONDITIONS -- to determine the impact
of the many medical and
non-medical factors on
populations and
communities.

ROBLEMS OF MEASUREMENT

eloping countries experience great problems in estab-
hing accurate indicators of health status because
 resources are limited and personnel and equipment are
short supply, (2) essential information collected at
 primary care level is often non-existent or grossly
dequate, (3) a large percentage of the population may
e <u>no</u> access to organized health care, so that information
lected within the organized health sector is limited
amount and accuracy, and (4) the rural areas may be so
lated that very little information can be obtained from
m. Therefore, where attempts are made to collect and
lish health data from developing countries, what
ally is presented are statistics from those segments of
 country where data <u>can</u> be obtained - the urban and
urban areas, and usually from the economically more
antaged part of the population.

HEALTH STATUS INDICATORS

A set of descriptive indicators has been evolved to
roughly estimate the health level of a community or
country. Some of these major indicators are:

Infant mortality rate
Life expectancy at birth
Crude death rate
Crude birth rate
Immunization rate
Age specific death causes
Incidence and prevalence of communicable diseases,
   which in many instances are the only reported ones
Resource assessment measures: hospital beds, clinic
   services, etc. per unit population
Manpower availability, doctors, nurses, auxiliaries,
   etc. per unit population
Present availability of potable water

These indicators are used singly or in combination to
provide a basis for health status assessment.

suspect that by now you have developed some personal
tions about the definition of health. Here is your
portunity to express these opinions.

At this point, using the information presented above
d your own knowledge about factors that influence health
d how they might be assessed, jot down a few words which
itique the World Health Organization definition of
alth ("a state of optimal physical, mental and social
ll-being, and not merely the absence of disease or
firmity"). Comment on both positive and negative aspects.

How do you think the applications and usefulness of
is defnition can be assessed in terms of the rich and
or countries?

SUGGESTED RESPONSES

*We recognize the difficulty in arriving at definitive state-
ments upon which we all would agree. However, perhaps you
included some of these ideas in your response.*

1. WHO DEFINITION OF HEALTH - (Some Positive Aspects): The
    definition focuses on health rather than disease. It
    aims at consideration of the "quality of life" rather
    than simply the physical health of the individual.

    (Negative Aspects): The definition is a utopian -
    probably far off - goal for which it is difficult to
    set objectives. In addition, it is difficult both to
    apply this concept and measure its results in terms of
    health status. Furthermore, this definition omits any
    consideration of whether health is a right or privilege.

2. DIFFERENCES IN APPLYING AND USING THE DEFINITION: In
    the rich countries data gathering is easier than in
    developing areas and there is information from a wider
    range of health indicators. However, there are factors
    accompanying an urbanized, industrialized life style
    which undermine the "quality of life" and make it more
    complex to maintain or achieve. In developing countries
    there are fewer data and resources with which to measure
    and confront health problems and much of the energy and
    concerns are focused on basic problems of survival,
    rather than on an "optimal" state of health and well-
    being. Nevertheless, there may be strong social and
    family relationships which add to the "quality of life"
    in these countries.

WORLD PATTERNS OF MORBIDITY AND MORTALITY *

r the two major population groups which have been class-
ied as "the rich and poor," measures of their health
atus reveal two distinct patterns of morbidity and mort-
ity. Although the following categorization is over-
neralized, it should provide you with an overview of major
alth problems characteristic of affluent and developing
untries.

most complex relationship exists between population dynamics
d patterns of morbidity and mortality. The shape of the
o contrasting population pyramids shown on the next page
e the result of intricate interactions between birth
te, morbidity and mortality. High birth rate in a
veloping country sets the stage for high infant mortal-
y while low birth rates in affluent countries are associated
ith a greater survival rate of infants. Thus, in developing
untries, the population percentages are heavily weighted
ward youth. Often fifty percent of the population is less
an 15 years of age - nearly twenty percent of the total
pulation is less than five years of age. How does it
ntrast with the population pyramid of most of the affluent
untries? Note that the rich countries have an older
pulation and a greater weighting toward the middle and
ter years of life.

_____

See also Unit I/2, "Worldwide Patterns of Disease"

POPULATIONS BY AGE GROUPS

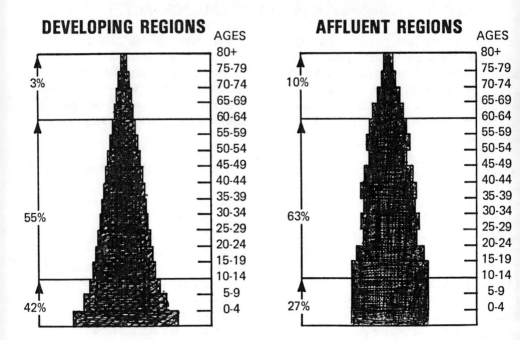

DEVELOPING REGIONS

AGES

	80+
	75-79
3%	70-74
	65-69
	60-64
	55-59
	50-54
	45-49
	40-44
	35-39
55%	30-34
	25-29
	20-24
	15-19
	10-14
	5-9
42%	0-4

AFFLUENT REGIONS

AGES

	80+
	75-79
10%	70-74
	65-69
	60-64
	55-59
	50-54
	45-49
	40-44
	35-39
63%	30-34
	25-29
	20-24
	15-19
	10-14
	5-9
27%	0-4

Note the high percentage of population below the age of 15 in developing regions as opposed to the more evenly distributed population across all age groups in the affluent regions.

If you look at Table 4 on the next page, you see that the developing countries show high birth rates in comparison to the affluent countries.

TABLE 4

DEMOGRAPHIC STATISTICS

or tries)	BIRTH RATE* (Per 1,000 Live Births)	DEATH RATE* (Per 1,000)	INFANT MORTALITY* (Per 1,000 Live Births)	GROWTH** RATE
gladesh	50	28	132	3.0
r Volta	49	26	160	2.3
stan	47	17	200	3.6
fluent tries)				
den	14	11	10	.2
nce	17	11	16	.8
.A.	16	9	18	1.0

rces: * U.S. & World Development Agenda for Action, 1975
         Overseas Development Council
         ** World Population Estimates, prepared by The
         Environmental Fund, 1975.

me of the developing countries of the world have population
owth rates which exceed 3.5% per year. (A population growth
te of approximately three percent per year means doubling
 the population in 23 years.) As a consequence, world
pulation is growing at an alarming speed. The affluent
tions in recent years are approaching or have attained zero
pulation growth - a state in which there is a balance be-
een birth rate and death rate, and migration in and out
 a country, so that population size remains numerically
able.

tice the differences in crude death rates. Whereas
ngladesh and Upper Volta approach rates of nearly 30
aths per thousand population each year, Sweden and France
ve a corresponding figure of only 11.

I/1, p. 23

In the developing countries, there are quite high infant
mortality rates* which range up to 200. In the affluent
countries, infant mortality rates have fallen as low as ten.

Not shown in Table 4, but another important indicator
because of its relationship to malnutrition and infectious
disease, is the death rate of children under the age of
five years.** In many of the developing countries, the
"under five" mortality rate is in excess of 350; that is to
say that more than one-third of all children born alive do
not survive beyond their fifth birthday. Under-five mortality rates in some affluent nations are lower than 20.
Maternal mortality rates in the developing countries also
remain high, as high as 50 or more deaths per 10,000 births,
while in the affluent countries, maternal mortality rates
have in some cases dropped to negligible levels - below
2 deaths per 10,000 births.

In the affluent countries, the reduction in childhood and
infectious diseases has resulted in a greatly decreased under
5 mortality and in an older population, with chronic
diseases and diseases related to aging. Life style, stress,
environmental decay, industrialization and pollution have
produced health problems rarely seen in the developing
world, where parasitic, infectious and childhood diseases
predominate. There, the synergism between infectious
disease and malnutrition plays a particularly important role.

---

*Infant mortality - deaths of children under one year of age
 per 1000 live births.

**Under-five mortality - deaths of children under five years of
 age per 1000 live births.

major exception to the above classification involves the
ople's Republic of China. This vast country, which contains
me 20% of the entire world's population, exhibits, in an
onomic sense, many of the features of the developing coun-
ies, but has apparently made an extraordinary transition
 its disease and health status patterns in recent years.
cause published data from the People's Republic of China
e just beginning to appear, it is still difficult to
sess and confirm the accuracy of statements made in this
spect. If you are interested in international health,
wever, you should follow developments in China, as they
y have important implications for morbidity and mortality
tterns as well as for health planning in all countries.

HEALTH CARE RESOURCES[*]

cope with health problems, the health care resources -
power, finances, and facilities of countries - vary
rmously. Because of low GNP in developing countries,
ancial resources available to health services are ex-
mely limited. From Table 5 on the next page, you can
 that the poorest of the developing countries expend
s than $1 per year per inhabitant on all government-
anced health services, and many of the other developing
ntries have a health expenditure in the range of $1 to
) per person per year. What is the corresponding figure
 the United States?

 capita government health expenditures in the developed
ntries actually exhibit a broad range from about $30 to
) per person per year. This type of figure is somewhat
fficult to interpret, because in different political
stems the government share of all health expenditures

For further discussion see Category V, "Health Care
Systems"

TABLE 5

HEALTH SERVICES (DOCTORS, HOSPITAL BEDS, GOVERNMENT EXPEND-
ITURES) IN FOUR COUNTRIES, 1965

	INDIA	BRAZIL	KENYA	USA
Population (millions)	469	81	9	195
Percent Population Urbanized (Cities of 100,000 or more)	9	30	6	28
Physicians/100,000 pop.	21	42	8	148
Hospital Beds/100,000 pop.	59	283	129	875
Government Health Expend-itures* ($U.S./per person/per year)	0.5	1.5	1.3	51

* Excludes non-Governmental Health Expenditures. Total annual
  per capita health expenditures in the U.S.A. are above $500

Source: Adapted from L. Corsa and D. Oakley, Rapid Population
        Growth, Johns Hopkins Press, 1971.

may be greater or less. For example, whereas there is a high
percentage of private health expenditures in the United States
the corresponding figure for the Soviet Union is very low.

Reflecting these economic indicators, developing countries
in general have a marked scarcity of trained health manpower
and of other health resources (hospital beds, clinics, drugs,
equipment, etc.). In addition to absolute scarcities, there
is often marked maldistribution of health care resources
between favored urban and relatively neglected rural areas and
between privileged and underprivileged population groups.

I/1, p. 26

ble 6 below reflects this disparity. Make a mental note
out the supply of physicians and hospital beds in the
pital cities of each of these three countries compared to
eir distribution throughout the rest of the nation.

TABLE 6

STRIBUTION OF DOCTORS AND HOSPITAL BEDS IN CAPITAL CITY
AND NATIONWIDE, THREE COUNTRIES (1964)

	POPULATION PER DOCTOR	POPULATION PER HOSPITAL BED	HOSPITAL BEDS PER DOCTOR
MAICA			
Nation	2,200	240	9.5
Capital City	840	90	9.3
Rest of Nation	5,510	540	10.0
NEGAL			
Nation	19,100	700	27.5
Capital City	4,270	280	15.2
Rest of Nation	44,300	920	48.0
AILAND			
Nation	6,900	1,200	4.5
Capital City	940	370	2.6
Rest of Nation	15,900	1,640	9.4

urce: Adapted from J. Bryant, Health and the Developing
World, Cornell University Press, 1969.

early, doctors and hospital beds are more plentiful in
e capital city than in the rest of the nation.

Another maldistribution of resources follows from an emphasis on hospital-oriented curative care which requires a great concentration of health manpower and equipment. In the affluent nations, even in the presence of a relative wealth of trained manpower and other health resources, there often exist similar major maldistributions, especially between urban and rural areas, and certainly between the economically advantaged and the disadvantaged.

WORLDWIDE OVERVIEW OF HEALTH AND DISEASE

It is important to emphasize that the gaps between the developing countries and the affluent countries are widening. Furthermore, most of the world's population must be counted among the poor. The population of the developing countries, if China is included, amounts to almost 70% of the world's population.

Furthermore, the world pattern of morbidity and mortality is heavily weighted towards the developing countries. Almost two-thirds of the world's current population live under rural conditions, although there is a progressively rapid shift of the population from rural to urban areas in both the affluent and the developing countries. With this displacement come problems of health that will continue to grow in importance - a combination of the infectious and parasitic disease of poverty together with the diseases of urbanization, industrialization and crowding and poor nutrition

Another important global demographic fact concerns the large number of the human population that is aged 0-5 or 0-15, especially in the developing countries. It is estimated that 60 million deaths take place annually on the globe, and of these, 30 million are children under the age of five years. It is estimated that one-half of these deaths (15 million) are the direct result of infectious disease, malnutrition, or a combination of these two. The important and complex

:eractions between infectious disease, nutrition and the cycle
rapid population growth cannot be overemphasized.

:r the last thirty or forty years there have been decisive
inges in the human condition which profoundly influence health.
: has been man's rapidly increasing technological control of
: environment, which has both positive and negative con-
ruences. On the positive side, man has developed powerful
rapeutic skills to treat disease, as well as bold tech-
ogies to improve water and waste disposal systems, while
the other side, the rise of human technology and its
itrol of the environment has led increasingly to environ-
ital decay and pollution, with negative health consequences.
: can cite as examples the hazards to life and health posed
the automobile, the problems of air and water pollution in
: industrialized countries, and problems of social disorgan-
ition and human violence occasioned by urban overcrowding.

ther important change has been the increasing interdependence
all human population groups, in part related to the rise
human technology. As the isolation between population sub-
ups and nations is disappearing, health problems and their
responding economic and political implications for one
ion or one population increasingly are being shared by all
ian population groups. For example, the potential for the
id spread of epidemics of infectious disease is made
sible by the modern system of transportation and commun-
tion between what were formerly quite isolated population
ups. In longer range terms, we must also recognize that
cycle of rapid population growth, high disease and death
es and acute nutritional shortages of the Indian sub-
tinent has some important political, economic and social
lications for the U.S. Such complex interrelated health
blems are not amenable to simplistic "single channel"
utions. They require an approach using a wide variety
professional and academic disciplines and skills working
hin an international framework. Society looks to health
fessions for much of the guidance and leadership in these
as. Involvement in international health activities gives

present and future health professionals the opportunity to observe firsthand that health problems are a reflection of not only economic, but also social, cultural and environmental conditions; and that their solution, or even improvement, will have to depend on the multidisciplinary cooperation of a wide variety of professional and academic disciplines and skills.

this point, review your work on Table 3 and add any other
pertinent information. Then compare the characteristics you
used to distinguish the affluent from the developing countries
with those provided in the synopsis on the next two pages.
Please add to your table any major items which you have
omitted.

TABLE 3

SYNOPSIS

CHARACTERISTICS OF THE AFFLUENT AND POOR COUNTRIES*

	AFFLUENT COUNTRIES	POOR COUNTRIES
I. ECONOMIC CHARACTERISTICS	High per capita gross national product Countries grouped as: over $1000/year (problem with comparisons to socialist countries)	Low per capita gross national product Countries grouped as: less than $150/year $150 - $450 $450 - approximately $1000
	High per capita health expenditures $30 - $400/year	Low per capita health expenditures, some less than $1/year, most $1 - $10/year
II. POPULATION CHARACTERISTICS	Longer history as independent nation states	Recent political independence; many were colonies of affluent nations until after World War I (major exceptions: Latin America and Thailand)
	In temperate zones of North America, Europe (including Russia) plus Japan, Australia, New Zealand, Israel, South Africa	Mostly in so-called "tropical" areas of Africa, Asia and Latin America
	Highly technological industrial development and mechanization of agriculture; capital intensive	Less development of industry and industrial technology; major part of population involved in subsistence agriculture; labor intensive
	Highly urbanized	High proportion of population rural (but recent trends to urbanization)
	Decline of traditional village and extended family organizational pattern Isolation and independence	Strong persistence of traditional village society

*These comparative statements are useful for descriptive purposes, but there are many exceptions when one compares individual countries.

TABLE 3

SYNOPSIS
CHARACTERISTICS OF THE AFFLUENT AND POOR COUNTRIES*

AFFLUENT COUNTRIES	POOR COUNTRIES
Older population	Population heavily weighted towards youth, often 50% of population less than 15 years of age, including nearly 20% of total population less than five years old
Low rates of fertility and birth; some countries nearing "zero population growth"	High rate of population growth (up to 3.5%)
Low crude death rates (7-10/1000 pop./year) and relatively long life expectancy at birth (up to 70+ years)	High crude death rates (up to 30/1000 pop./year) and relatively short life expectancy at birth (as low as 30-40 years)
Low infant mortality rates (as low as 10/1000 live births)	High infant mortality rates (up to 200/1000 live births)
Low under five mortality rates (as low as approximately 20/1000 births)	High under five mortality rates (up to 350/1000 live births)
Low maternal mortality rates (as low as 2/10,000)	High maternal mortality rates (up to 50/10,000)
Mortality and morbidity patterns emphasize: diseases related to aging chronic disease in an older population health problems related to environmental decay and pollution, accidents and trauma related to industrialization (especially the automobile)	Mortality and morbidity patterns emphasize: infant and young children infectious and parasitic diseases, malnutrition in early childhood and its synergy with infectious diseases
Relative wealth of trained manpower and other health resources though often major geographic and specialty maldistribution	Marked scarcity of trained manpower and other health resources

These comparative statements are useful for descriptive purposes, but there are many exceptions when one compares individual countries.

SUMMARY REVIEW

Having completed the material in this unit and developed
your table of characteristics to differentiate the affluent
from the developing countries, again consider the six
questions posed at the beginning of the unit. Our responses
follow each question. You may add your comments or notes
in the spaces provided.

1. Characteristics of the rich and poor countries: how
    would you define "development?"

    "Development" is a multi-variable term which relates
    most closely to economic and broader "quality of life"
    factors. As summarized in Table 3, the world's nations
    fall roughly into "poor" (sometimes called "less devel-
    oped:) and affluent groups.

2. Can we define "health?" If no, why? If yes, how?

    Health can be defined if you are willing to consider
    the WHO definition of health as "a state of optimal
    physical, mental and social well-being, and not merely
    the absence of disease or informity." But this definition
    is difficult to understand in an operational sense. It
    reflects, however, one measure of the "quality of life"
    and thus is closely tied to "development."

What factors influence health?

The health of individuals and communities is influenced, not only by biologic, but also by non-biologic factors including economic, political and socio-cultural ones, especially as they are reflected in the environment in which we live.

How can we measure and compare these factors?

Indices have been developed by which to measure and compare health factors. Although no group of these measures gives a complete assessment of "health" or of "quality of life," nevertheless these factors are useful as approximate indices.

5. What are the major world patterns of morbidity and
   mortality?

   Differences in the amount and distribution of available resources (wealth), as well as global differences in
   life styles are responsible for two major patterns of
   morbidity and mortality in the world. One reflects the
   population/nutrition/infectious and parasitic disease
   syndrome most prevalent in poor populations. The other
   reflects the effects of industrialization, urbanization
   and environment pollution and decay that are most closely
   tied to affluent life styles.

6. What resources do countries have available to deal with
   health problems?

   Different countries and different population groups
   within nations have widely differing amounts and kinds of
   resources such as finances, trained personnel, facilities
   and supplies - with which to meet their health problems.

If you have gotten these messages out of this unit, you may
wish to focus more specifically now on the epidemiologic
patterns of affluent and developing countries (Unit I/2).
However, if areas were unclear or prompted questions which
were not answered, you should review the pertinent sections
of the unit and discuss major points with your instructor.

ADDITIONAL REFERENCES

yant, J. Health and the Developing World. Cornell
iversity Press, Ithaca and London, 1969.
   A fundamental analysis of the health status of the
   world's poor, based on broad statistics as well as on
   the author's extensive experience.

ller, R.B. Operating Manual for Spaceship Earth. Simon
 Schuster, New York, 1970.
   An architect's and planner's view of development in a
   multidisciplinary sense.

rdal, G. Asian Drama. Inquiry Into the Poverty of Nations.
ntheon, New York, 1968.
   An extensive (2 volumes) and detailed presentation of the
   social problems, including health, facing the developing
   countries, using Southeast Asia as the source for many
   examples, but valid for most of the developing world.

rdal, G. Challenge of World Poverty: A World Anti-Poverty
)gram in Outline. Pantheon, New York, 1970.
   As the title implies, this is an imaginative and innovative approach to development, based on the extensive
   experience and thought of the author.

rd, B. (Lady Jackson) The Rich Nations and the Poor Nations.
 W. Norton & Co., New York, 1962.
   A short, concise presentation of the dilemma the world
   is facing in relation to the widening gap between the
   affluent and the "developing countries.

Wolstenholme G., and O'Connor M. Health of Mankind.
Spottiswoode, Ballentyne & Co., London, 1967.
   A symposium dealing with the broad overview of health
   and disease on a global basis.

The Assault on World Poverty, with a preface by R.S.
McNamara, Johns Hopkins University Press, Baltimore, 1975.
   In sections on Rural Development, Agricultural Credit,
   Land Reform, Education and Health, proposals are made to
   combat world poverty in a multidisciplinary way.

Health Sector Policy Paper. World Bank, 1975.
   A description of programs and methods which the World
   Bank plans to use in the health field.

Health by the People. Edited by Kenneth W. Newell.
WHO Geneva, 1975.
   A collection of articles by a multi-national group of
   health care planners dealing with the specific problems
   of third world countries.

World Eco-Crisis. Edited by D.A. Kay and E. Skolnikoff.
University of Wisconsin Press, Madison, 1972.
   A broad range collection of articles on successes of and
   constraints to international programs dealing with the
   environmental problems.

UNIT I/2 WORLDWIDE PATTERNS OF DISEASE

BY

STEPHEN C. JOSEPH, M.D., M.P.H.

OBJECTIVES

Each of the units within Category I is aimed at illustrating the dramatic differences that can exist in health patterns among various populations. More specifically, this unit is intended to examine worldwide patterns of disease. After you have completed the material you should be able to:

1. Describe the historical disease patterns that have been exhibited throughout centuries of development by affluent Western countries,

2. Identify the predominant disease patterns in the world today and distinguish differences among selected population groups on the basis of biologic, geographic/environmental and sociocultural factors.

3. Explain major contemporary disease patterns both geographically and historically.

INTRODUCTION

Epidemiology (from the Greek roots "epi" = upon or on, "demos" = the people) is the study of diseases in groups of people, rather than in individuals. The epidemiologist thus analyzes characteristics of diverse human populations. These characteristics may be: biologic (such as age, sex, and genetic characteristics), geographic/environmental (such as the size and physical lay-out of human communities or climatic and topographic factors), and sociocultural (such as patterns of social, economic and political organization, and behavioral traits and customs).

The notion of a community or a population group as the "unit" of investigation for health care is central to our epidemiologic perspective. Just as we can apply qualitative and quantitative methods to the study, prevention, and treatment of disease in individual patients, so can we apply analogous methods to

study, prevention, and treatment of disease in population
ups.

thermore, just as disease patterns and disease characteris-
s vary between individuals and at different stages of any
ividual's life-cycle, disease patterns and characteristics
o vary among different population groups and at different
torical periods within a community or other human popula-
n. These geographic, cultural, and historical variations
be very useful in helping us to understand important
ationships between human communities and disease so that
can support individual and group characteristics which
or health, and combat those which favor disease.

our purposes in this unit, three epidemiologic concepts
uld be kept in mind:

A human population (such as a community or nation) can
be viewed as the unit of study, prevention, and treatment of diseases, just as an individual can be so viewed.

Patterns of disease in human populations vary with, and
also influence, the biologic, social and environmental
characteristics of population groups. These patterns
can be scientifically described and measured.

Major patterns of disease vary, not only geographically
(through space - across communities, cultures, nations),
but also historically (through time).

WORLDWIDE DISEASE PATTERNS

ist of major diseases causing morbidity and mortality
ay must certainly reflect the following categories of
ease:

cer,

ectious and parasitic diseases,

malnutrition,

cardiovascular diseases,

accidents and trauma.

If we are to select from these categories the three most
important disease patterns producing severe morbidity and
mortality in 1975 for an affluent country such as the United
States we would list cardiovascular disease, cancer, accidents
and trauma. Were we making the same assessment for the year
1775, however, our selections would have been different (see
Table 1).

TABLE 1

CENTURY	USA, CANADA OR U.K.	PERU, ZAIRE OR PAKISTAN
c. 1975	cardiovascular disease cancer accidents and trauma,	infectious and parasitic diseases malnutrition accidents and trauma
c. 1775	infectious and parasitic diseases accidents and trauma malnutrition	infectious and parasitic diseases malnutrition accidents and trauma

Please pay special attention to the most important causes of
mortality in 1975 for the poor countries listed on the table
above. After first noting the historical disease patterns of
the affluent countries and then considering the likelihood that
there will be geographical differences in disease patterns today (especially between affluent and poor countries), the following supporting rationale can be given:

1. The chronic degenerative disease patterns that typify the
    aging affluent population of the U.S.A., Canada or the
    United Kingdom in 1975 will not be as evident in poor
    countries which have much younger populations.

Malnutrition and infectious and parasitic diseases are presently not the leading causes of mortality in affluent countries, but they used to be, and still are the major causes in poor countries.

The position of accidents and trauma in both the affluent and poor countries relates to the detailed nature and causes of accidents and trauma in the two situations. The rich, heavily industrialized countries show a predominance of industrial and motor vehicle accidents, and of trauma related to mechanized agriculture. The poor countries show a predominance of trauma, including (especially) burns occurring during traditional agriculture and household pursuits. The potential for large scale industrial accidents and environmental disasters (man made disasters) is greater in the rich countries with complex interdependent technologic infrastructures. The occurrence of death and injury in "natural" disasters (earthquakes, floods, wind storms) is greater in poor countries because of less-resistant shelter and man made infrastructure, and less resources available for disaster response.

Two centuries ago the major causes of diseases and death in the affluent countries were close to those of poor countries today. Furthermore this "traditional" pattern has been common to most human groups throughout history. Despite increased knowledge and technology, many of today's impoverished countries have not achieved improved levels of nutrition, a more sanitary environment, or adequate prevention and curative treatment against infectious diseases. As a result, the major patterns of disease in poor countries have probably not changed much over past centuries. It is even possible that malnutrition was actually less prevalent in former centuries in some traditional societies before population pressure increased to current levels without concomitant rise of agricultural output. The rapid urbanization and conditions of extreme poverty found today in many developing countries foster infectious and parasitic diseases and malnutrition, because of crowding of populations under conditions of poor sanitation and other environmental hazards.

With this epidemiologic introduction to global disease
patterns, let's now look more closely at diseases patterns
across time (historical epidemiology) and across space
(geographic epidemiology).

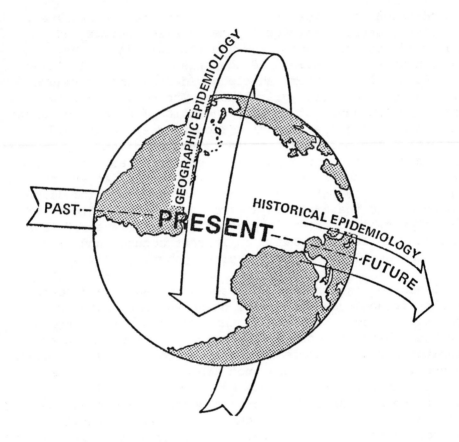

.ve periods can be identified in the affluent West that
)rrelate with changing epidemiological patterns: (1) tra-
itional agrarian society, (2) urbanization and the industrial
evolution, (3) the sanitary revolution and the rise of
ffluence, (4) the biomedical revolution and the age of tech-
ology, and (5) the post-industrial state. These periods
epresent general trends and the dates shown should be
.ewed as illustrative rather than exact.

aditional Agrarian Society (through the 17th Century)

he prevailing patterns of morbidity and mortality were the
:raditional" patterns, i.e. a predominance of deaths in
arly childhood (under age 5) caused by the interaction of
.lnutrition and infectious diseases. Communicable diseases,
specially of the respiratory and gastrointestinal systems
ere uncontrolled, epidemic diseases were rife, and diseases
ich as malaria were endemic in large parts of Europe and
rth America.

banization and the Industrial Revolution (17th-late 19th
enturies)

he period saw rapid urbanization, the development of industrial
echnologies (and mass employment), and major strides in
ansportation, communications, and trade (including the
cploitation of foreign colonies). However, particularly
irly in this period, these changes were accompanied by per-
stent mass poverty, poor nutrition, unsanitary environmental
nditions, and crowding of urban populations. In many
stances, death rates rose, especially in the new urban
vironment. The ever present diarrheal and respiratory
seases were augmented by new importations of epidemics
ch as yellow fever from foreign commerce, and tuberculosis,
ich became a scourge of major proportions among the urban
or.

The Sanitary Revolution and the Rise of Affluence (mid-19th to mid-20th Century)

With increasing social and economic equity, and technological development, the affluence of the West was reflected in pro-gressive sharp declines of death rates, especially in what were the "traditional" disease categories. Safe water supplie and sewage disposal improved nutrition and decreased contamina tion of foods, safer housing and working conditions, mass education - all these produced remarkable improvements in heal well before specific advances in medical therapy were availabl

The Biomedical Revolution and the Age of Technology (early mid-20th Century through the present and foreseeable future)

There have been pervasive medical advances in the last forty years beginning with the introduction of new vaccines and the sulfonamides in the 1930s, the proliferation of antibiotics after penicillin, the fruits of clinical pharmacology and biochemistry, the achievements of surgery and organ transplan-tation, and the development of psychoactive drugs. All these measures have created a health technology so powerful and so pervasive in the West that most people (including medical students and younger physicians) do not realize how recent these developments are, and how much improvement in human health had been accomplished previously without them.

On the other hand, the biomedical advances of recent and current history have brought two new perspectives to our thinking about disease patterns: (a) as "old" diseases are reduced in frequency and severity, "new" diseases move in to take their places, creating a shift of patterns whereby the causality of mortality patterns change, but man's ultimate fate remains the same; and (b) as the power of the biomedical technology has increased, so the dangers and illness-producing effects of its application have also increased. The hazards of biomedical technology were highlighted, for instance, in a study of university hospital patients in the early 1960s in which almost one-third of all patients admitted to a medical

I/2, p. 8

rvice suffered a significant medically untoward event while
the hospital - drug errors or reactions, injuries from tests
therapeutic procedures, complications of surgical or medical
eatment, etc.

e Post-Industrial State (present and probable future)

e progressive shift of morbidity and mortality towards de-
nerative diseases and diseases of aging shows every sign of
ntinuing. These patterns, in an "aging" population pyramid
d accompanied by a massive increase in the cost of applying
e biomedical technology at all ages, are increasingly ques-
ned about ethical as well as cost-effectiveness issues
uching on almost all we do in medicine. There is also the
arge that the affluent societies are becoming "medicalized"
to a dependence upon prescription and non-prescription drugs.
is concept, and the broader concerns of "iatrogenesis" and
edical nemesis" may be over-reactions to the dilemmas and
fects of modern biomedicine and modern life itself, but they
e indicators of perceived or real defects in some of the
nsequences of the biomedical revolution.

e biomedical technologic and post-industrial periods have
en accompanied by the rise of a newly-important spectrum
 diseases related to man's increasing ability to pollute
d despoil his environment. Biologic, chemical, and radio-
gic health hazards accompany industrial and technologic
velopment. Alterations of natural environments and human
bitats create new social and psychological stresses which
ve the potential of precipitating psychosocial disorders
 individual and group scales. Finally, the ever-present
man potential for violence and destructiveness is now
tched with the technologic capacity for mass destruction
 civilian populations on a global scale.

I/2, p. 9

A Review

Clearly, the epidemiology of disease patterns in affluent Western countries has changed considerably within a time span of less than 300 years. On the basis of what you have read, please respond to the questions which follow:

Table 2 presents disease specific mortality rates at selected intervals over a hundred year period in New York City.

TABLE 2

DISEASE SPECIFIC MORTALITY RATES FOR NEW YORK CITY

NEW YORK CITY	1870	1890	1910	1930	1950	1970
DEATH RATE FROM:						
Tuberculosis (General Population per 100,000)	396.1	361.9	210.5	73.1	29.4	4.9
Diarrheal Disease (Under Five-Years per 100,000)	3380	2060	1167	157	14	7
Measles (General Population per 100,000)	26.9	37.6	16.4	2.2	less than 0.05	None
Expectancy of life at birth (years)	N.A.	N.A.	47.4	57.9	68.1	70.1
Infant Mortality Rate (per 1,000 live births)	277.2	262.1	125.6	57.2	24.8	21.6
Maternal Mortality Rate (per 10,000 live births)	252.0	139.4	59.0	54.3	7.6	4.6

SOURCE: ANNUAL REPORTS OF NEW YORK, BUREAU OF HEALTH STATISTICS AND ANALYSIS, NEW YORK CITY.

N.A. = not available

I/2, p. 10

To what do you attribute the decrease in mortality rates between 1870 and 1930?

The table shows a further drop in selected death rates by 1950 and 1970. How do you explain these reductions?

1.   (a) *The decrease in mortality was due largely to improved nutrition and to the sanitary revolution which began around the turn of the century. While improvements in diet, water purification and waste disposal were starting to be felt in 1890 (with lower death rates from tuberculosis, diarrheal disease and the general infant mortality rate per 1000 live births, but <u>not</u> in deaths from measles), by 1930 all indicators show drastic reductions in mortality.*

    (b) *The mortality figures in the later years are due to advances occurring in the biomedical revolution, e.g. antibiotics and sophisticated intravenous fluid therapy after 1945, improved medical and surgical obstetrics, measles vaccine following 1965.*

The health status data below are descriptive of a
ciety type.   (Note: 1976 rates for the U.S. are given
 parenthesis.)

ude death rate = 30 deaths per 1,000 population per year
   (US = 9 deaths per 1,000)
ude birth rate = 40 births per 1,000 population per year
   (US = 15 per 1,000)
te of Natural Increase = 1 percent per year (US = less than
   1.7 percent per year)
fant mortality rate = 150 deaths under 1 year of age
   per 1,000 live births (US = 17)
der 5 death rate = 250 deaths per 1,000 population aged
   0-5 years (US = 20)
ternal mortality rate = 60 per 10,000 live births (US =
   4 per 10,000)

ich of the following type of society is described by
ese data?

____(a) an affluent society in the post-industrial state
        of development

____(b) a traditional agrarian society

____(c) a society of growing affluence following the
        sanitary revolution

2. *(b) A traditional agrarian society is the appropriate response, because a pattern of high fertility balanced by high mortality, especially mortality in early childhood, suggests a society endangered by infectious diseases and malnutrition. (This same pattern also would tend to characterize small hunter-gatherer populations and the urban population of both former and present times in what are now called "developing" countries.)*

There are a number of health care situations in affluent post-industrial states that have given rise to questions both of ethics and/or cost effectiveness of what is done in medicine. Several examples are cited below:

1. Without a clear definition of death it is difficult to discern the limits of medical responsibility in the efforts to preserve and prolong life.

2. From one to three percent of all U.S. primary school children are labelled "hyperactive;" about half of these children receive drug therapy for behavior modification. The effectiveness, hazards and long-term effects of this therapy are uncertain.

3. Despite the high cost and large number of surgical operations done for tonsillo-adenoidectomies and hysterectomies, clear and medically agreed upon guidelines of indications for, and effectivess of, both procedures do not exist.

4. Although the advances in medical technology have made possible very sophisticated forms of treatment, this same health technology has given rise to a whole range of new illnesses. In addition, modern health technology is responsible for significant side effects.

e mortality patterns which have accompanied these advances
technology are shown in relation to Canada (Table 3).

TABLE 3

MAJOR CAUSES OF MORTALITY, CANADA, 1971

se	No. of Deaths	% of All Deaths	Predominant Ages
:HAEMIC :RT DISEASE	48,975	31.1	40 and over
:EBROVASCULAR :EASE	16,067	10.2	65 and over
:PIRATORY DISEASES :ND LUNG CANCER	15,677	10.0	Under 1 year and 55 and over
:OR VEHICLE AND ALL :THER ACCIDENTS	12,031	7.6	All ages
:CER OF GASTRO- :NTESTINAL TRACT	7,947	5.1	50 and over
:CER OF THE BREAST, :TERUS, AND OVARY	4,816	3.1	40 and over
:EASES SPECIFIC TO :HE NEWBORN	3,299	2.1	Under 1 week
:CIDE	2,559	1.6	15 to 65
:GENITAL ANOMALIES	1,967	1.3	Under 1 year
TOTAL	113,338	72.1	
. DEATHS IN CANADA, 1971	157,272	100.0	

RCE: Lalonde, Marc, A New Perspective on the Health
of Canadians, 1974

As Western biomedical technology expanded, and as the advances in public health began to be applied to poorer countries and colonial areas, there were similar dramatic decreases in morbidity and mortality to those seen in the West during and following the Sanitary Revolution. However, the changes were nowhere nearly as profound or widespread, given the persisting poverty of the colonial setting, nor were there broadly distributed systems by which to reach the population with clinical care. In many, if not most, colonies, the application of all these measures was geographically quite limited, usually for the purposes of either ensuring the health of resident colonizers, and/or of promoting and assisting (through the prestige and appeal of health services as well as their results) military, economic, and religious colonizing objectives. Thus, especially in rural areas and in newly-created and existing urban slums, the major patterns of disease and death persisted. In other areas death rates fell but fertility rates remained high (or increased, with improved nutritional status), thereby resulting in the rapid population growth amidst poverty and scarce resources that continues through present times.

In the poorer countries of the world, especially the newly independent nations of Africa and Asia, the traditional disease patterns still prevail, although the health care systems have been modelled after those of the West. Furthermore, even though there have been many local demonstrations and experiments at developing locally appropriate innovations in health care systems emphasizing mass applicable, low technology-dependent, low cost, health measures that can reach rural and urban populations, only a few countries such as the People's Republic of China, North Vietnam, and Tanzania have adopted national health policies that move unequivocally in these directions (among other countries whose early efforts should be followed carefully by those interested in these issues are Papua New Guinea and Mozambique).

e major patterns of diseases in today's world have already
en described. These patterns are in large part biologically
termined but have been influenced by economic and political
velopments, as well as by cultural patterns. There are
so important geographic characteristics that influence
e expression of disease.

making geographic epidemiologic comparisons, factors of
ography and climate are the most important considerations
art from those determined by human biology and behavior.
viously, a parasitic disease that depends for part of
s life cycle on aquatic snails and fishes (as does
histosomiasis) will be found in geographic proximity to
dies of water which have the appropriate physical charac-
ristics to favor development of the parasites and host
ncluding the biologic and behavioral characteristics of
n, snails, and fish!).* Similarly, a disease produced by
organism that is inhibited by certain climatic conditions
uld not be expected to be found with great frequency, if
all, in settings where those climatic conditions prevail.

ctors associated with unusual disease frequency

rich interplay of biologic, geographic/environmental, and
ciocultural characteristics, many of which are, if at all,
ly poorly understood, produces the detailed pattern of
sease as it varies from community to community and nation
nation. Bladder cancer, for example, is especially
evalent among Egyptian farmers. As another unusual disease
ttern, African children suffer in large numbers from
rkitt's lymphoma. Why? Unfortunately, we do not know
e certain etiology of these diseases or the etiologies of
e other malignancies listed below. Nevertheless, we can

For a further discussion of the schistosome life cycle,
see Unit III/4, "Ecological Determinants of Health Problems."

partially explain the high frequency of these and other
diseases by noting some of the associated biologic,
geographic/environmental, or sociocultural factors.

MALIGNANCY AND POPULATION DEMONSTRATING UNUSUAL FREQUENCY	ASSOCIATED FACTORS
Bladder cancer in Egyptian farmers	high rates of chronic bladder infection with parasite - Schistosoma hematobium
Oropharyngeal carcinomas in Thailand - especially in market women	widespread betel-chewing, with irritating lime (calcium oxide) added to betel nut and leaf wrapper plus other species and additives
lung cancer (bronchiogenic carcinoma) in American and European males	Cigarette smoking Respiratory pollutants in industrial areas
Esophageal carcinoma in Iran, along Caspian Sea	? dietary factors ? genetic predisposition No clear understanding of factors
Burkitt's lymphoma in African children	Relationships with specific conditions of temperature and humidity; ? Association with insect vector and/or malaria Probable causal chain related to EBVirus

While a definitive understanding of the "cause" of each of
these cancers awaits further developments in the field of
molecular biology, these examples show how associated factors
can shape disease patterns.

y is shigella dysentery more prevalent in an urban setting
Mali (West Africa) than in rural eastern Wyoming?

ter having compared some of the environmental, behavioral
d biologic features of the populations of each location,
we have done below, it is easy to see that Bamako affords
more hospitable environment than eastern Wyoming to the
read of shigella dysentery.

TABLE 4

ME FACTORS INFLUENCING THE OCCURRENCE, SEVERITY, AND SPREAD
SHIGELLA DYSENTERY IN TWO HUMAN POPULATIONS

	(Eastern Wyoming, U.S.A.) Temperate-Zone Rural Area	(Bamako, Mali, West Africa) Tropical-Zone Urban Area
ssociated ctors		
ologic	-Older Population -No herd immunity -Well nourished pop. -Generally healthy pop. -Etc.	-Younger Population -No herd immunity -Poorly-nourished pop. -Many intercurrent diseases Etc.
ographic/ vironmental	-Dispersed pop. -Safe water supply -Safe excreta disposal -Adequate household water available -Climate unfavorable to bacterial growth	-Crowded population -Unsafe water supply -Unsafe excreta disposal -Household water scarcity -Climate favors bacterial growth -Etc.
cio/Cultural	-Inhibits fecal oral transmission, (handwashing, etc.)	- favors fecal-oral transmission

If you dismissed the idea that Shigella dysentery might exist as readily in eastern Wyoming as in Mali, you may have done so after considering not only the geographic differences between the two locations, but also the historical development of disease patterns in the wake of social, economic and cultural change. Put another way, you might expect coronary artery disease to be a greater health problem in eastern Wyoming than in Mali. Why?

At this stage in the development of your epidemiologic perspective, an important question concerning the historical and geographic comparison between rich and poor countries should have occurred to you. If so, it probably sounds something like this:

Does the historical development of disease patterns of the West presage quite similar evolutionary disease patterns in poor countries? Are the "diseases of poverty" the diseases of the past for our human species, and are the "diseases of affluence" the diseases of the future?

ere are arguments both for and against an answer of "yes"
 the question. Assuming a "yes" answer, briefly list
ır arguments for and your arguments against such a response
 the question on the previous page:

₹:

AINST:

en compare your thoughts with ours which appear on the
 lowing page.

Suggested Responses:

FOR	AGAINST
- *Historical similarity of the traditional pattern of the West with the pattern in poor countries today*	- *Profound cultural differences in the affluent and poor countries*
- *"Development" may produce patterns of urbanized and industrialized societies in all countries*	- *"History" in the late 20th century is quite different from "history" in the late 18th and 19th centuries*
- *The increasing interdependence of human populations, and man's increasing control of the environment (for good and for ill), create a trend towards homogeneity of all human populations*	- *In particular, the pressures of population growth and food and other resource scarcity make it a new and unique situation*
	- *Also, the availability of modern health technology and future biomedical research gains make the situation of the future for the poor countries quite different from the situation of the past in the affluent countries*

UNIT REVIEW

As a final exercise, to demonstrate how you can employ the material presented in this chapter, look at the exercise table on the next page. The cells of this table allow for description of the world in the year 2075, and of the health and disease pattern of rich and poor countries under two different sets of circumstances. Fill in the Table with your own prognosis - be both as detailed and creative as you can. Your prognosis in this table sets the parameters of the work for the next century for those interested in international health! A set of responses with which you may compare your own is shown on the completed table on pages 24-25.

TABLE 4 - THE WORLD'S HEALTH IN 2075

Alternative Scenarios	Rich Countries	Poor Countries	Outcome
increasing disparities in health, continued rapid population growth and food shortages, and increasing environmental pollution			
more equitable distribution of health, stabilized population growth and environmental protection			

I/2, p. 23

Suggested Response:

ALTERNATIVE SCENARIOS	RICH COUNTRIES
If, increasing disparities in wealth, continued rapid population growth and food shortages, and increasing environmental pollution: then probable-	*Accelerated "diseases of affluence" up to the point where environmental decay, and global chaos secondary to events in poor countries, cause "system breakdown", followed by a renewed importance of the "traditional" pattern of "diseases of poverty" - even in the currently "rich" countries*
If, more equitable distribution of wealth, stabilized population growth, and environmental protection:	*Cyclical pattern of "diseases of affluence, with technologic and social solutions to one set of health problems producing the conditions for the rise of relative and absolute importance of a "new" set of problems. Probable areas of high importance in 2075 include:* *1. Physical and psychosocial problems of aging and "increased leisure" in the general population* *2. Environmental hazards (trauma, toxins, radiation)* *3. "Diseases of Medical Progress" (complications of medical and surgical and transplantation therapy)*

POOR COUNTRIES	OUTCOME
Tightening spiral of food/ population/health constraints. Increase of "diseases of poverty" to a scale unprecedented in human history	*War* *Famine* *Epidemics* *Possible self destruction of "spaceship Earth"*
Gradual shift towards patterns of rich countries, but unlikely that the underlying causes of traditional infectious/nutritional disease patterns will be overcome by 2075. More likely, the result will be an intermediate position.	*Whether the health and equity "gaps" between rich and poor countries will narrow significantly and to what extent, depends more upon nutrition, population, and international economic and political balances, than upon the development and transfer of health technology*

You should plan to discuss any questions or other points of note with your instructor. Also, you might wish to consult some of the additional references which follow.

ADDITIONAL REFERENCES

1. Dubos, Rene, _Mirage of Health_, A Doubleday Anchor Book, Garden City, New York 1961.

2. Fuchs, Victor, _Who Shall Live?_ Basic Books, New York 1974.

3. Illich, Ivan, _Medical Nemesis: The Expropriation of Health_, Marion Boyars London, 1975.

4. Lalonde, Marc, _A New Perspective on the Health of Canadians, 1974_, Information, Canada, Government of Canada.

5. McDermott, Walsh. _Modern Medicine and the Demographic/ Disease Pattern of Overly-Traditional Societies: A Technologic Misfit._ J. Med. Education 41: (Suppl.) 137-162

6. McKeown, Thomas, _Medicine in Modern Society_, George Allen and UNWIN Ltd., London, 1965.

UNIT I/3: THE HEALTH OF THE WORLD'S CHILDREN

BY

STEPHEN C. JOSEPH, M.D., M.P.H.

CONTENTS

OBJECTIVES

"Children" and "childhood" are general terms; usually we don't stop to think whether they mean the same thing in all situations. Nevertheless, while no child is truly "typical," the life profiles of children may be strikingly different throughout the world, especially between rich and poor societies. The purpose of this unit is to examine the health of children from an international perspective.

After completing the unit you should be able to:

1. Explain, in a general way, who are the world's children.

2. Discuss major child health problems, using health status indices that have been developed.

3. Recognize the range of growth and development patterns of children in various societies.

4. Explain selected health problems of infectious disease, malnutrition, behavior and accidents in terms of the social environment and growth patterns of children.

INTRODUCTION

Who are the world's children? In 1970, the world's children comprised upwards of 1.5 billion people (out of almost 4 billion people on earth) (See Table 1). They are heavily concentrated in the poorer countries of the world. In fact, about

TABLE 1

TOTAL AND CHILDHOOD POPULATION, "MORE AND LESS DEVELOPED" REGIONS, c. 1970

	"MORE DEVELOPED REGIONS"	"LESS DEVELOPED REGIONS"	WORLD TOTAL
Population, all ages (millions)	1090	2544	3634
Population, aged 0-5 years (millions)	98	432	532
Population, aged 0-15 years	293	1068	1361
Population, aged 0-5 years as % of total population	9	17	15
Population, aged 0-15 years as % of total population	27	42	38

Source: Adapted from World Bank, _Trends in Developing Countries_, 1973.

80% of the world's children live in poor countries, almost three-quarters of them in rural settings. Furthermore, children under 5 years of age account for 15-20% of the total population of these countries. By way of contrast in the more developed regions, the majority of children live in urban environments, often in small families.*

Severe but quite typical health problems to which the world's children are exposed are presented in the four case histories given below. You may wish to make some notes about these problems, or to underline significant points as you read them. Later, at the conclusion of this unit you will be asked questions about the health patterns they represent.

Amadou is the third current survivor of 7 children born in a family of farmers in an isolated village in Mali. At 16 months of age, he is markedly underweight, with swollen feet and legs, and he suffers from repeated bouts of diarrhea. His mother is five months pregnant, and abruptly weaned Amadou two months ago, increasing his diet of millet gruel. Amadou's village has a Koranic school; the nearest government school is 20 miles away in a larger village, where there is also a poorly-equipped dispensary. No motorable roads link the two villages.

Beatrice is a 7 year old child in a farm family of five just outside a city of 250,000 in Britain. She is blind, as a result of a viral infection her mother contracted in early pregnancy, before a vaccine against this virus became generally available. Beatrice receives specialized

---

*Actually, there is also a strong trend towards urbanization (especially in migration of young adults) in many developing countries. Within the next 25 years, it is possible that the urban population of most of South America will out-number the rural population, and the relative proportion of rural populations in Asia and Africa will almost certainly diminish in comparison to urban population.

edical care through the National Health Service, and attends
school for multiple-handicapped children in the city. She
ad a moderately severe congenital heart defect corrected
urgically at age 5, and has abnormally short stature and
orderline-normal intelligence.

arlos is a 10-year old "street boy" in Bogota, Colombia.
hough small in size, he describes himself in "excellent
ealth but always hungry." Carlos lives by his wits, forag-
ng in the streets and sleeping in the alleys. His "family"
s the loosely constructed pack of street children that
amed him - he recalls no other antecedents. Carlos is
lliterate, unimmunized, and appears in no set of government
r international statistics.

elma is a 13 year old black girl in Chicago. Her face is
adly scarred as a result of a kerosene stove fire that
urned down the one-room shack in Mississippi where she and
er parents lived until she was three years old. Delma lives
th her grandmother, her mother, and three siblings aged 4
o 10. Her mother has just lost her factory job and is
everely depressed. Delma has announced that she "doesn't
nt to waste time in that school anymore, because I need to
lp take care of the family." Her IQ, recently tested at
chool, is 140.

WHAT IS CHILD HEALTH?

ildhood is the period of greatest growth, development, and
aturation of the human organism. This period involves a
radual and progressive transition from the total dependency
f intra-uterine existence to relatively independent function
s an adult. Elements of dependency include biologic (food,
elter, protection from various hazards), psycho-social
ntellectual and emotional development), and cultural
socialization and education, economic). The beginning of
ildhood is clearly marked by birth, but the "end" of the
riod is diffuse and not clearly bounded. For medical
rposes (especially in the affluent countries), childhood

is assumed to end at age 15 or 16, at a point where physical growth and sexual maturation have passed watersheds. However, in most affluent countries, economic and educational dependency may continue well into third and even fourth decades of life.

Usual age at marriage is another rough indicator of the end of childhood in many societies; this may vary by more than a decade (12 or 13 years to mid-20s or beyond) in different societies and for individuals within a given society. Puberty, economic independence, mastery of adult work roles, age of legal consent, military obligations, and many other parameters are useful, but inexact, measures of childhood's end in various societies.

For purposes of comparison and classification, childhood has been divided into several age periods. These age periods are useful in describing growth, developmental and socializing processes. They include infancy, secotrancy, early childhood, school age, and adolescence. In most affluent countries, "pediatrics" usually concerns itself with the health of children from birth through mid adolescence (15-16 years of age). In striking contrast, the attention of child health workers in most developing countries is primarily focused on children less than 5 years of age. Since, in both groups of countries children under 5 account for about 1/3 of all children, this difference in perspective is not based on proportional differences within the childhood population. It relates, rather, to differences in prevailing patterns of health and illness in the two settings.

Let's look more closely at these age periods, as well as the health and illness problems that they entail. We will divide them into two groups: One, the age periods and health problems of children under five; and two, the development of children between the ages of 5-15.

e sum of health hazards posed by the dependency and initial
posure to biologic and physical agents in the environment
at a maximum during the first two years of life. Thus,
fant and secotrant mortality are sensitive reflections of
population's ability to protect its existence.

fancy

fancy extends from birth to the end of the first year of
fe. This is the period of most rapid growth and develop-
nt in the entire life-span and also the period of greatest
pendency (with the possible exception of the dependency of
itical illness and/or extreme aging).

cotrancy

is term is not very frequently employed, but repre-
nts an important concept for understanding death and
sease patterns of children in poor countries. The secotrant
 the child in the <u>second</u> year of life, i.e. between 1 and
years. In addition to continued rapid (though decelerating
om infancy) physical growth and psycho-social development,
o all-important processes take place during this period,
rticularly in traditional societies.

Weaning and Its Nutritional Consequences - Shortly before
or during early secotrancy, breast milk is often withdrawn
as the major or only nutritional source. Though some
supplementation with other foods may have been started in
early infancy, it is particularly in the second year of
life that progressive and/or cumulative nutritional
deficits become apparent after the child is weaned.

Increased Contact with the External Environment - The
secotrant's increasing locomotor and other (e.g. hand-to-
mouth) exploratory activities bring him/her into much
greater contact with the external environment and its
multiple infectious and traumatic hazards.

EARLY CHILDHOOD

Early childhood usually means the period from birth to the
fifth birthday (expressed as age 0-5 years). In many
societies, this period is one in which the child's major
sustained contacts do not pass far beyond the home and family
environment. This period precedes formal education of the
child in peer groups. There are three important exceptions
to this generalization: (1) in social settings where mothers
carry their children with them at almost all times (e.g. many
West African farming cultures), there is early and sustained
contact of young children with non-family adults and childhood peers, (2) for working parents in such diverse countries
as China, USSR, and Israel, communal child care facilities are
commonly found, (3) in the U.S.A. and other industrialized
states, there is a trend towards increased day-care and pre-
school activities.

Some Questions About Health Patterns in the Under Fives

Available data about disease and death statistics usually
concern rates in infancy (0-1 years) and/or early childhood
(0-5 years).

Study Table 2 on the next page.

1. What does table 2 tell you about the comparative health
    problems of young children in affluent and poor countries?
    Jot down some of your thoughts below.

DEMOGRAPHIC DATA FOR AFFLUENT AND POOR COUNTRIES
TABLE 2

	BIRTH RATE* PER 1,000	INFANT MORTALITY* PER 1,000 LIVE BIRTHS	AGE 1-5** MORTALITY RATE	
Affluent Countries			Males	Females
United States	15	17	17.9	17.7
Sweden	13	9	9.5	9.4
Japan	19	11	12.1	11.8
Poor Countries				
Chad	44	160	Not available	
India	35	139	Not available	
Guatemala	43	79	40.8	38.4

*Source: 1976 World Population Data Sheet, Population Reference Bureau, Washington, D.C.

*Source: United Nations Demographic Yearbook, 1974.

2. What two major health factors would account for the differing infant and early childhood mortality rates between affluent and poor countries?

    (a)

    (b)

1. *The table illustrates the dichotomous child health pattern of affluent and poor countries. Poor countries are characterized by high birth rates and high infant and early childhood mortality rates, while richer countries tend to have lower birth rates but higher child survival rates. High birth rates add increased pressure to the problems of scarce resources in poor families and populations. High birth rates also reflect short birth intervals within a family. Rapid repetition of pregnancy in poor families is reflected in earlier weaning and poorer nutrition of the existing infant/secotrant. Further, the secotrant whose mother is pregnant or nursing a new infant probably is at a higher risk and is less protected from the hazards of the environment than the child who is weaned at a later date.*

2. *Thus, these differing mortality rates* reflect: (a) Nutritional determinants, and (b) Infectious disease determinants.*

---

* Infant mortality rate (deaths occurring before first birthday per 1,000 live births) provides information about infection, but by itself does not sufficiently assess nutritional status or some environmental hazards; Under-5 mortality rates (deaths occurring before 5th birthday per 1,000 children in this age group) does include the high nutrition and infectious disease risks of the 2nd year of life but also include a later period (late 4th and the 5th year) when many of the most critical nutritional and infectious watersheds have been passed. Thus, neither index is by itself ideal for comparing childhood mortality. For a fuller discussion of health indices, see Unit II/1, "Assessment of Health Problems and Resources."

at are the "specific" diseases most responsible for the
gh rates of disease and death in young children in poor
untries?   Table 3 should give you an idea. Look particu-
rly at the statistics for diarrheal diseases, pneumonia
d malnutrition.   (Not represented in the table, but another
jor killer in many countries, is tetanus.)

JOR CAUSES OF DEATH IN THE UNDER FIVE (PERCENTAGES OF DEATHS)

TABLE 3

	IMESI NIGERIA 1957	LUAPULA ZAMBIA	NORTH SUMATRA	PUSAN SOUTH KOREA
arrheal seases	12	18	25	15
eumonia	12	10	11	9
lnutrition	12	16	26	14
laria	8	15	8	3
ooping ugh	8		2	4
asles	8	13	7	16
berculosis	5		6	8
allpox	5			
emia		7	5	
her, mostly onatal	30	21	10	24
tal number all ildren	-	340	1,282	1,036

urce: Taken from Morley's Pediatric Priorities in the
veloping World, London: Butterworths, 1973. Reprinted
th permission.

In a classical description of the major traditional patterns of childhood morbidity and mortality, McDermott coined the phrase "diarrhea-pneumonia complex." This concept is extremely important, because it recognizes the fact that:

1) Gastro-intestinal and lower respiratory diseases are the most important infectious diseases causing high early childhood mortality, and

2) Most of these infectious episodes are caused by viral and bacterial organisms against which we either do not now have specific preventive or therapeutic agents, or did not have such preventive and therapeutic agents during the time periods when morbidity and mortality fell precipitously from these causes in the West.

Questions:

Figure 1 graphically demonstrates the predominant causes of infant mortality over a period between 1900-1930.

A. Where would you say these data were gathered?

(1) _____ The World
(2) _____ The USSR
(3) _____ Hong Kong
(4) _____ The Philippines
(5) _____ New York City

PREDOMINANT CAUSES OF INFANT MORTALITY
FIGURE 1

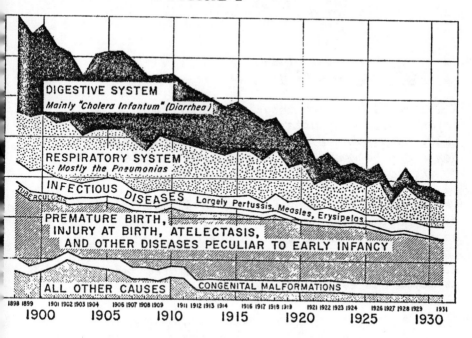

What was the reason for your answer to question A?

A. (1) _____ The World
    (2) _____ The USSR
    (3) _____ Hong Kong
    (4) _____ The Philippines
    (5) XXXX New York City

B. New York City is the only location listed in which the
    infant mortality pattern had improved so greatly by
    1930. Nevertheless, the pattern was replicated by
    Hong Kong between 1950-1970 and, in fact is similar
    to that of many developing countries today.

    The point of this exercise was to illustrate the magnitude
    of infectious diseases (especially diarrheal diseases)
    as a cause of death, even in our own country in the past.
    Compare, for example, the age specific death rates from
    diarrhea (Table 4) between New York City and the Punjab
    at different historical junctures.

AGE-SPECIFIC DEATH RATES FROM DIARRHEA
TABLE 4

PLACE (time)	RATES 100,000	
	0-11 months	1-4 years
New York (1911)	5603	399
New York (1961)	45	2.4
Punjab, India (1959)	3446	312

Source: Gordon, et al. Am. J. Science, 245: 345 (1963)

Note that New York City had a higher rate in 1911 than the
Punjab in 1959.

Unfortunately, accurate statistics on early childhood
mortality (under 5 years of age) in developing countries
are scarce. However, in those countries with the highest

ath rates in early childhood, the following is a useful rule
thumb: 180 of each 1,000 infants born alive die in the
rst year (infant mortality rate); 150 die in the next 4
ars (early childhood mortality rate); 75 of these die be-
ween the ages of 1 and 2 (second-year mortality). Thus, a
ird of all live-born children in countries with the highest
ildhood death rates die by the fifth birthday.

en comparing progress in developing countries, you might
ep in mind the following:

) the most sensitive indicator of improving nutritional
   status is the second-year mortality;

) the most sensitive indicators of improved control of
   infectious disease (especially the diarrhea-pneumonia
   complex) are the infant and second-year mortality rates;

) "under-fives" mortality (early childhood mortality) is
   a good surrogate measure for indicating the status of
   the all-important synergistic relationship between
   infection and malnutrition in a population.

ring the age periods of infancy through early childhood, a
scussion of world health problems must stress the relation-
ip between malnutrition and infectious disease. However,
 later age periods the major health problems are more
osely linked to psychosocial and cultural adjustment.

. CHILDREN BETWEEN AGES 5 AND 15

hool Age

is period roughly covers the ages 5 or 6 through 11-12,
rresponding in the U.S. to primary school (including junior
gh school). Much of this period corresponds in develop-
ntal terms to the "latent period," and a rough marker of
s end is puberty.

Adolesence

This period, roughly from puberty to the late teens, covers
the more-focused transition to adulthood - in physical,
emotional, economic, and life-role terms. Key characteristics
of this period (such as strong peer-group identification,
ambivalence towards authority, rebellion, pronounced self-
consciousness, heightened idealism, etc.) have been described
mainly based on observations of Western populations; they
should be applied cautiously in non-Western and especially
traditional subsistence cultures where age-grouping, early
progressive assumption of adult economic tasks and roles,
world-view and values systems, etc., may be considerably
different in character and timing. Biologically, the
maturational changes of adolescence (especially skeletal
maturation and development of secondary sexual characteristics,
are relatively constant across the human species, as are the
progressive heterosexual interests in adolescence which
normally culminate in mating and marriage. However, some
variation is inherent in all human biologic and social behavior. By way of example, the average age of menarche in
North America has decreased by roughly a half-decade (from
15-16 years of age to about 11 years of age) in the past
two centuries. This is thought to relate principally to
improved nutritional status, and indeed age at menarche in
less well nourished populations is later, in clear refutation
of the myth of early puberty in "tropical" populations.

The relationship betwen malnutrition and intellectual
development is nowhere near as clear as that between
malnutrition and physical growth. It is certain that poor
nutrition has indirect effects upon a child's ability to
learn (examples: inability to concentrate or perform well in
school due to hunger, lassitude due to anemia, etc., or
dropping out of school to earn money needed for food, etc.)
but the question of whether malnutrition in infancy and early
childhood produces irreversible intellectual damage is not

...t settled - this crucial issue should be followed closely
... all students interested in the health of children, for it
...s the most important implications for attempts to break
...e cycle of poverty, ill-health, and malnutrition.

NUTRITION, INFECTION, GROWTH AND DEVELOPMENT

...ny formats have been developed for expressing the "normal"
...owth patterns of children. The most commonly used system
...ots increase in weigth or height against increase in
...ronologic age for a "standard" population of "normal"
...ildren at various ages. Using the concept of a normal
...stribution, the 3rd from heaviest (or tallest) child among
...0 "normal" children of age x (say, 14 months) would fall
... the 97 percentile, the 3rd from lightest (or smallest)
... the 3 percentile, and the median child on the 50 percentile.
...e can readily see the potential for argument about what
...nstitutes a "standard" or "normal" population, especially
...en data derived from one socioeconomic setting are utilized
...r another. However, what is unequivocally clear is that
...fants and children with under-nutrition and high prevelance
... infectious disease display a significantly poorer growth
...rformance than children of the same ethnic group who have
... better nutritional and health pattern.

... practice, the weight and height percentiles most often used
... a reference base are the Boston growth charts. Because
...e growth performance of children in most of the developing
...rld has been found to be significantly less than the Boston
...tandards," however, a commonly used modification has been
...vised which sets a range of "normal" weights for children
... developing countries that spans the distance between the
...d percentile and 50th percentile of the Boston curve (or
...her curve designed for a well-nourished European population).
...gure 2, on the next page, illustrates the range of weights
...r "normal" child growth.

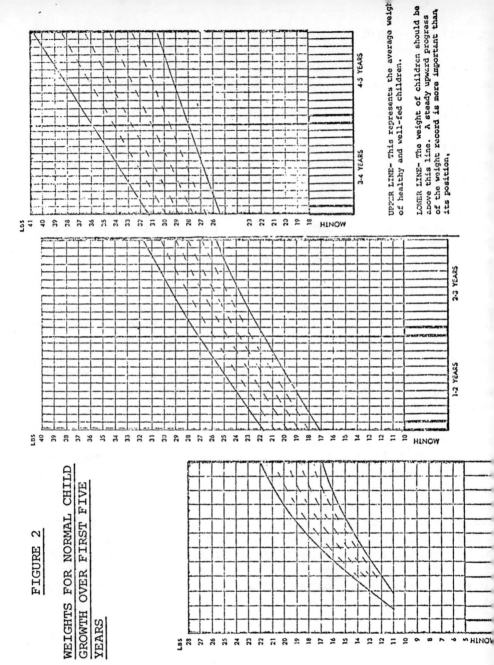

FIGURE 2

WEIGHTS FOR NORMAL CHILD
GROWTH OVER FIRST FIVE
YEARS

UPPER LINE- This represents the average weight
of healthy and well-fed children.

LOWER LINE- The weight of children should be
above this line. A steady upward progress
of the weight record is more important than
its position.

other words, a child in most developing countries can be
nsidered to be of adequate weight for a given age if his/
r weight is equal to at least the 3 percentile weight (which
self is two standard deviations from the median weight) of
ll-nourished children in Boston or Europe of the same age.
ny systems have been described for classifying types and
grees of malnutrition, using variations of the above
scribed systems. Weight, height, weight-height ratios,
m or thigh circumference, skin-fold thickness (a measure
fat) all have particular advantages and disadvantages.
vertheless, despite the difficulties (insufficient data
ailable, difficulty of collecting adequate data, problems
defining a universal versus a local reference standard,
oblems of defining "normal" and "optimal" growth in
fferent societies and populations) the growth chart,
pecially the weight chart, is the most powerful tool we
ve for assessing the nutritional status of a childhood
pulation.

e weight chart is also the most powerful tool we have for
sessing the growth, nutritional status, and life and
alth status of the individual child in a developing
untry. The growth curve, sensitive to nutritional and
fectious insults, has been graphically described by Morley
"the road to health." A line representing the child's
ight at various ages, compared to the lower and upper
oundaries of the road," is much more important than a
ngle determination of weight at one age, and is a convenient
y to demonstrate to mothers the importance of adequate
trition and its relationship to growth and health.

A Quick Summary

Figure 3 shows the weight curve of a child in a rural village in Asia. **FIGURE 3**

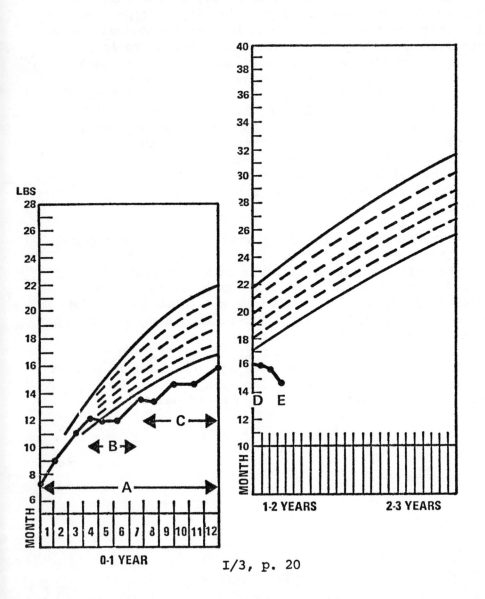

I/3, p. 20

om the information available on the weight chart on page 20, is possible to plot the impact of the following series of ents in a child's growth and development:

Period Point	Age	Event
	0-12 months	Breast-fed
	5-6 months	Several bouts of diarrhea and malaria
	8-12 months	More diarrhea and respiratory infections
	12 months	Weaning, followed by progressive malnutrition
	15 months	Measles, followed by rapid progression of malnutrition

By the end of 15 months the child in the preceding example is severely endangered by the results of the synergistic relationship between malnutrition and infectious diseases. As you can see from Table 5, a state of continued nutritional deficiency often is associated with death or early childhood.

TABLE 5

Nutritional Deficiency as Associated Cause of Death Under 5 Years of Age (Excluding Neonatal Deaths) by Underlying Cause Group in 13 Latin American Projects

UNDERLYING CAUSE GROUP	TOTAL DEATHS	NUTRITIONAL DEFICIENCY AS ASSOCIATED CAUSE	
		No.	%
All causes......	21,951	10,349	47.1
Infectious and parasitic diseases	12,598	7,667	60.9
Diarrheal disease	8,770	5,331	60.8
Measles	2,103	1,311	62.3
Other	1,725	1,025	59.4
Nutritional deficiency	1,163		
Diseases of respiratory system	4,469	1,435	32.1
Other causes	3,721	1,247	33.5

Source: Puffer and Serrano, Patterns of Mortality in Childhood, PAHO, 1973.

DIFFERENCES BETWEEN THE AFFLUENT AND THE POOR

MORBIDITY AND MORTALITY

In the materially wealthy societies of the affluent countries, the morbidity and mortality patterns of childhood are dramatically different from those of the poor countries. With the elimination of high morbidity and mortality from infectious diseases brought about by improved nutrition, safe water and waste disposal, general increase in living standards and, later, by immunization and medical therapeutics, the remaining major causes of childhood mortality in affluent countries tend to be accidents and violence (now the first cause of death in Americans between the ages of 1 and 45, followed by malignancies, and congenital diseases, both genetic and from complications of pregnancy. Suicide is currently the second leading cause of death at age 15-24.)

Significant morbidity and mortality from infectious diseases after infancy in a given society, and any occurrence of malnutrition (except for that associated with metabolic or anatomic dysfunction leading to decreased food intake or poor absorption) is now taken to provide an indicator of the presence of disadvantaged groups within the society, who do not share equally in the economic or health benefits available to the majority.

Review

Table 6 (see pages 24-26) contains the profile of a male child (age 11) living in a suburb of Boston. Undoubtedly, the life of this child contrasts in many ways with the life of a child born in a rural area in a poor country. Complete the profile for the 11-year old rural child living in a village in Mali.

TABLE 6

PROFILES OF 2 MALE CHILDREN – 11 YEARS OF AGE

Profile Characteristics	Suburban child, Industrialized society (e.g. suburbs of Boston, U.S.A. 1977)	Rural child Traditional agricultural society (e.g. village, Mali, West Africa, 1977)
No. of living siblings/no. of ever-born siblings	2/2	
Feeding and nutritional patterns	- artificial feeding (bottle-fed) – birth – 1 year - diet high in protein, refined sugars, and saturated fats - adequate to excessive caloric intake	
Formal education	- pre-school and kindergarten - primary school to (current) 5th grade	

I/3, p. 24

Major routes of learning of parental, gender, and social roles	- television (has observed approximately 8,000 hours) - school - parents (father communtes to office in city 20 miles away; contact with mother almost constant until age 5 - peers and siblings - indirect emulation of adult social and economic roles through "play"
Capsule disease history (From parental recall, in physician's phrasing)	- infant colic - childhood diseases. chickenpox and mumps, ages 7 & 8 - dental caries - fractured tibia due to auto-bicycle accident

I/3, p. 25

TABLE 6 (cont'd)

Major contacts with health professionals	- hospital delivery; obstetrician - well and sick-child care; pediatrician (x 14 until age 1; average x 4 yearly since then) - dentist (yearly since age 6) - school psychologist regarding reading difficulty
Aspirations regarding adult occupation/ (actual outcome)	- "I want to be an astronaut and go to the moon, or play first base for the Boston Red Sox" (office worker - middle management in large corporation in Los Angeles, California)

SUGGESTED RESPONSES: While there are many acceptable ways in which you could have completed your profile, certainly your description of the Malian child should have contained striking contrasts to the profile of the child living in an affluent Western country.

Our SUGGESTED RESPONSES are presented on the next two pages.

TABLE 6

Profiles of 2 Male Children -- 11 years of age

	Surburban child, Industrialized society (e.g. suburbs of Boston, U.S.A. 1977)	*Rural child, Traditional subsistence society (e.g. Village in Mali, 1977)*
No. of living siblings/ no. of ever-born siblings	2/2	4/7
Feeding and nutritional patterns	— artificial feeding (bottle-fed) - birth - 1 year —diet high in protein, refined sugars, and saturated fats —adequate to excessive caloric intake	— *breast fed to age 14 mont undernourished in second year of life* — *diet low in protein* — *diet low in refined sugar and saturated fats*
Formal education	—pre-school and kindergarten — primary school to (current) 5th grade	—*attended village school f 3 years functionally illiterate*
Major routes of learning of parental, gender, and social roles	—television (has observed approximately 8,000 hours) —school —parents (father commutes to office in city 20 miles away; contact with mother almost constant until age 5 —peers and siblings —indirect emulation of adult social and economic roles through "play"	—*parents and extended fami (3 generations in same household)* —*peers and siblings* — *direct emulation and earl assumption of adult-type economic and social roles (household work, tending goats, farming tasks, etc beginning at age 6-7)*

TABLE 6   (cont'd)

apsule disease istory	infant colic	- *severe diarrhea and malaria attacks "many times"*
From parental recall, n physician's hrasing)	childhood diseases. chickenpox and mumps, ages 7 & 8	- *significant under-nutrition and anemia, age 1½ - 2 years*
	dental caries	- *measles, age 1½*
	fractured tibia due to auto-bicycle accident	- *whooping cough, age 2*
ajor contacts with ealth professionals	- hospital delivery; obstetrician	- *home delivery; traditional midwife*
	- well and sick-child care; pediatrician (x 14 until age 1; average x 4 yearly since then)	- *illness care by grandmother and village traditional healers*
	- dentist (yearly since age 6)	- *treated by nurse at health center 10 miles from village for measles pneumonia*
	- school psychologist regarding reading difficulty	- *vaccinated versus smallpox by mobile team, age 5*
Aspirations regarding adult occupation/ (actual outcome)	- "I want to be an astronaut and go to the moon, or play first base for the Boston Red Sox"	- *"I will be a farmer in my village"*
	- (office worker - middle management in large corporation in Los Angeles, California)	- *(farmer in the village where he was born)*

Regardless of whether a country is rich or poor, infancy provides a period where infectious diseases (gastro-enteritis, respiratory infections, meningitis) remain major causes of mortality, especially in the case of premature infants. However, with the striking advances of the past decade in the care of premature and unusually small infants, infant mortality rates have fallen to levels of approximately 10 per thousand live births in some countries, almost 20 <u>times</u> lower than some developing countries! At these contemporary low levels (10 - 30 per thousand live births), infant mortality rates provide another useful international comparison of (a) socioeconomic equity or homogeneity across the entire population and (b) associated equity of access to all available measures of preventive and curative medical care.

We might speculate that the "irreducible minimum" of infant mortality (severe congenital- anatomic and/or metabolic - anomalies incompatible with life, prematurity so severe as to be incompatible with pulmonary or renal function, major accidents at delivery, etc.) is around 5 - 7 deaths per thousand live births. <u>But</u>, the emergence of new techniques of prenatal diagnosis and genetic screening, and the advances just coming over the horizon in prenatal treatment and per-haps genetic engineering, as well as liberalized approaches to abortion, may well reduce this "irreducible minimum" even further within your professional lifetime, to perhaps 3 - 5 infant deaths per 1,000 live births.

PATTERNS OF FAMILY STRUCTURE

Whether one considers the nutritional needs and infectious hazards of children in the developing countries, or the lifestyle and environmental hazards of quite different kinds that face children in the affluent countries, the physical and emotional health of children is extremely dependent upon the adult social structures that surround them in their daily lives, and which heavily shape their growth and development.

I/3, p. 30

most societies, the most important biologic and social
interactions occur within the "nuclear family" (mother,
father, and children). However, in many traditional societies, especially in village-based cultures, the nuclear
family is strongly embedded in an "extended" or "joint" family
in which multiple generations (grand-parents and sometimes
great-grand-parents, parents, children and extended kinship
lines (uncles, aunts, cousins, etc.)) interact closely on a
daily basis, sometimes sharing the same dwelling. These
traditional family patterns have important effects in the
sharing of child-caring roles, the transmission of child-care
knowledge and practices across generations, the adoption of
personal, family, and social roles by children, and the
continuity of "belonging" to a lineage of persons and often
a place.

Industrialization and urbanization in the West (and increasingly in developing countries) has made major changes in
these patterns. Migration to urban areas, urban anonymity,
and industrial-society job mobility have loosened, and in
some cases shattered, the extended family and home-place
bonds of traditional society. These dislocations of traditional family patterns bring multiple and important hazards
to the physical and emotional health of children. In the
United States, for example, there are vast changes occurring
in the family structure. Perhaps you can speculate about
the implications for child development of each of these
three trends currently taking place in the United States.

Marked increase in <u>single-parent families</u>. For example,
one-quarter or more of all American children currently
live in single-parent families. Much of our child-rearing
lore and practice is based on the two-parent nuclear family.
Further, rising divorce and re-marriage rates have markedly
increased the numbers of children who experience "serially-
multiple" parenting.

2. Marked increase in full and part-time employment of married women (and/or female parents) in careers <u>outside</u> the home. This trend likewise creates new demands in child-rearing and child health not a part of our "traditional" culture.

3. Increase in alternative lifestyles, group marriage, communal living, etc. Despite the experiences in other countries (Israel, People's Republic of China, etc.) with alternative/communal systems of child-raising and child care, child health advocates will have to make major adjustments in their conceptual framework to cope with the effects of this trend.

It is noteworthy, however, that, in the affluent countries, besides the severe morbidity and mortality caused by accidents and malignant disease, attention has turned to behavioral disorders (school - and life-adjustment problems, disturbed parental-child relationships; enuresis, constipation, and other psychosomatic symptoms, etc.) as a major activity of pediatrics. The "anticipatory pediatrics" combination of dealing with life-adjustment problems of families with children <u>and</u> the preventive measures of well-child health supervision and immunization provide, in addition to the care of non-life threatening episodic illness (mostly minor respiratory, gastrointestinal, and skin infections and minor trauma), form the large bulk of the practice of pediatrics today in the affluent countries.

A Summary Review

A. Throughout the world in impoverished areas, the major hazards for child growth and development are nutrition and infection. Several points in particular should be stressed:

1- Protein-energy malnutrition affects tens of millions of children in the developing world, whose growth potential is certainly reduced and whose potential for intellectual development may also be affected.

In combination with infectious disease, with which there
a synergistic relationship, malnutrition is the most
portant cause of child mortality in the world, accounting
r perhaps one-quarter of all the world's annual deaths,
d half the deaths under 5 years of age.

Assurance of adequate nutrition in the early childhood
pulation would by itself do more to reduce high early
ildhood mortality than any other single measure or
mbination of measures, including provision of safe water
pplies and control of communicable disease.

Promotion of prolonged (well into the second year) breast-
eding, combined with adequate nutritional supplementation
solid foods from 4-5 months of age onwards, is crucial to
equate and safe nutrition of infants and secotrants in
verty populations in developing countries. Irresponsible
mmercial advertising campaigns that seek to promote mass
ttle feeding of infants in developing countries represent
health hazard of the highest order.

In many of the affluent countries, biomedical technology
s invited an expansion of child health concerns into
rontier areas." Some of these areas are:

Access to high-quality, readily-available, continuous,
d personalized health services (preventive, curative, and
habilitative) for all families and children in our society,
a cost that the society and its members can afford.

Advocacy for "children's rights" in terms of educational,
onomic, political, and social factors which affect their
alth (examples: improved education available to all
ildren, protection against child abuse, protection against
vironmental hazards such as lead paint, etc.).

Understanding of and effective action upon the "lifestyle"
d behavioral elements which are currently most important
disease-producing factors in our society (examples: safety

I/3, p. 33

and accident-prevention, anti-smoking education, prevention of adult atherosclerosis by dietary and exercise habits begun early in childhood, etc.).

4- Improved diagnosis and management of chronic <u>diseases and disability</u>. If visual and auditory deficits are included, it is estimated that one-third of American children have some major or minor chronic health problem. Orthopaedic and metabolic dysfunctions, developmental retardation, and reading and learning disabilities, are among the most important types of chronic disabilities in the U.S. childhood population. Many of the children with disabilities, though minor, could benefit from improved methods of diagnosis and management; many are associated with secondary behavioral emotional dysfunction.

5- New advances in prevention, diagnosis, and management of currently "untreatable" or only partially-treatable diseases. Advances in such areas as childhood cancer, diabetes, cystic fibrosis, sickle cell disease, and other less-prevalent medical and surgical conditions are important, and will provide both direct and indirect benefits.

6- Discovery of "new diseases," prevention and management of "diseases of medical progress" (iatrogenic disease), and fundamental advances in our understanding of the biology of children and illness; these areas will always provide a frontier for scientific inquiry and progress.

A UNIT REVIEW

arlier, you were presented the case histories of four child-
en and asked to examine their health problems, especially in
erms of the various health patterns that each child represents.
ow by way of a final review, you are being asked to apply what
ou have learned about the disease patterns of the world's
hildren. For each of the four children described, on the
ext page, please do the following:

    (a) Assess the present health level from the informa-
        tion given , and
    (b) Try to predict the status of the child five years
        from today.

Amadou is the third current survivor of 7 children born in a
family of farmers in an isolated village in Mali. At 16
months of age, he is markedly underweight, with swollen feet
and legs, and he suffers from repeated bouts of diarrhea.
His mother is five months pregnant, and abruptly weaned Amadou
two months ago, increasing his diet of millet gruel. Amadou's
village has a Koranic school; the nearest government school
is 20 miles away in a larger village, where there is also a
poorly equipped dispensary. No motorable roads link the two
villages.

atrice is a 7 year old child in a farm family of five just
tside a city of 250,000 in Britain. She is blind, as a
sult of a viral infection her mother contracted in early
egnancy, before a vaccine against this virus became
erally available. Beatrice receives specialized medical
e through the National Health Service, and attends a
ool for multiple handicapped children in the city.
e had a moderately severe congential heart defect corrected
gically at age 5, and has abnormally short stature and
derline-normal intelligence.

Carlos is a 10-year old "street boy" in Bogota, Colombia. Though small in size, he describes himself in "excellent health but always hungry." Carlos lives by his wits, foraging in the streets and sleeping in the alleys. His "family" is the loosely-constructed pack of street children that named him - he recalls no other antecedents. Carlos is illiterate, unimmunized, and appears in no set of government or international statistics.

Delma is a 13 year old black girl in Chicago. Her face is badly-scarred as a result of a kerosene stove fire that burned down the one-room shack in Mississippi where she and her parents lived until she was three years old. Delma lives with her grandmother, her mother, and three siblings aged 4 to 10. Her mother has just lost her factory job and is severely depressed. Delma has announced that she "doesn't want to waste time in that school anymore, because I need to help take care of the family." Her IQ, recently tested at school, is 140.

Hopefully, in your responses you integrated major features of child health and growth patterns such as those presented here.

1. (a) <u>Amadou</u> *exhibits the classical malnutrition-infectious disease pattern of early childhood in traditional rural societies. Furthermore, his poor nutritional status is exacerbated by abrupt weaning and short interval before the birth of the next child. As a mid-secotrant, Amadou is at the peak of risk in a setting where preventive and therapeutic public health and medical measures are virtually unavailable.*

   (b) *Amadou subsequently contracted measles at age 17 months. He had severe pneumonia and protracted diarrhea, but survived the acute phase of the disease. However, three weeks after the rash disappeared, full-blown symptoms of kwashiorkor became apparent, and Amadou died at age 19 months.*

2. (a) <u>Beatrice</u> *has a congenital disease acquired through secondary maternal viral infection whose etiology, pathogenesis and prevention have been elucidated in the past thirty years. Although the disease is preventable by vaccination (of the mother before reproductive age) it involves a complex multi-system pathology treated by sophisticated and expensive medical technology. The "life-adjustment" aspects of this chronic disease will cause Beatrice to seek the services of special institutions designed to help the multiple-handicapped.*

   (b) *At age 12, Beatrice is an active girl just beginning adolescence. She has become adept at Braille; previous estimates of "borderline normal" intelligence have been revised upwards. Her aspiration is to become a teacher of visually handicapped children, and it is probable that she will be able to function* well as an independent adult. Beatrice's mother expresses increasing concern about the child's "differentness" (blindness, short stature) as she enters adolescence; Beatrice herself is enthusiastic about entering the public high school in her community in two years.

(a) _Carlos_ reflects the social/economic/health linkages of poverty, especially in a situation of rapid and disorganized urbanization, as well as isolated rural settings. Carlos is evidence that the health problems of children extend far beyond definitions of physical illness.

(b) At age 12, Carlos sustained a fractured femur when hit by a car in a narrow street. He was hospitalized, treated, and upon recovery "placed" in an orphanage where his nutritional, shelter, and educational "problems" were addressed. After three weeks, Carlos climbed out a second-story window and returned to the streets. At age 14, he was stabbed in the abdomen during a quarrel. After treatment at the municipal hospital, a court ordered Carlos returned to the orphanage. This time he fled on the second night after his arrival. A bewildered young social worker, seeking to understand why Carlos would leave the security of the institution, was told by a colleague "you can't do anything with people like that. They're different."

(a) The case of _Delma_ illustrates the point that accidents are a leading cause of morbidity and mortality in childhood, and further that they, along with infectious disease, occur disproportionately among minority and poverty groups in affluent countries.

(b) Delma was persuaded to stay in school by the combined efforts of her grandmother and a teacher whom Delma admired. The family was able to hold together, *despite economic difficulties and mother's recurrent depression. Delma's sister, now 14, is pregnant and out of school. Delma is 18 and graduating near the top of her high-school class. She has a scholarship to a nearby university, and hopes eventually to go to law school. Delma has had two skin grafting operations on her face, done at a nearby municipal hospital where she is followed intermittently in the "plastic clinic"; these have produced minimal cosmetic improvements.*

Perhaps in examining these four case histories you were struck by the differences in the health of the world's children, especially when comparing rich and poor societies. Maybe you recognized that what can be considered as a problem or state of health in one society cannot be thought of in the same light within another setting. Is it possible to group certain attributes as child health in a universal sense? If so, what would constitute such an international concept of child health? Consider the following:

1. An optimal standard of child health in any society consists in the fulfillment by each child in that society of his/her physical, intellectual and social potential, given that the child-nurturing and protecting resources (at whatever level available in that society) are equitably distributed across all its members.

2. The potential of individuals, as influenced by the society in which they live, should be constantly expanding (with increasing advantages and decreasing disadvantages) under conditions of equitable distribution and growth of resources and wealth.

You may also wish to consult some of the references we list for more information about international child health, and/ or discuss it with your instructor.

ADDITIONAL REFERENCES

Coles, Robert, Migrants, Sharecroppers, Mountaineers: Volume II of Children of Crisis, Little Brown and Company, Boston, 1971.

Coles, Robert, Children of Crisis: A Study of Courage and Fear, Little Brown and Company, Boston, 1967.

The Dag Hammarskjold Foundation. Action For Children. Towards an Optimum Child Care Package in Africa. The Dag Hammerskjold Foundation, Uppsala, 1975.

Haggerty, R.J., Roghmann, K.J. and Pless, I.B.: Child Health in the Community, Wiley Interscience Series, New York, 1975.

Morley, David, Paediatric Priorities in the Developing World, Butterworths, 1973.

Puffer Ruth Rice., Serrano, Carlos, V.: Patterns of Mortality in Childhood. Pan American Health Organization, Pan American Sanitary Bureau, Regional Office of the World Health Organization, 1973.

Williams, Cicely, D.; Jelliffee, D.B.: Mother and Child Health: Delivering the Services, Oxford University Press, London, 1972.

UNIT I/4: DEVELOPMENT AND THE ALLOCATION OF HEALTH RESOURCES

DIETER KOCH-WESER, M.D., PH.D.

CONTENTS

OBJECTIVES

The overall purpose of the units in Category One is to provide you with a worldwide overview of health and disease. Here, the intention is to focus on methods and resources as well as constraints throughout the globe.

Problems are looked at from the point of view of social medicine, rather than economics. The focus is on the interaction between society and health, that is the way health -- and its absence -- influences society and how society deals with health problems. After completion of this unit you should be able to:

1. Name and generally describe the difficulties involved in allocating resources to improve health throughout the world.

2. Explain the interdependency of curative, preventive and rehabilitative medical services.

3. Describe the possible composition of a health team and diagram a three level health care organization.

4. List and describe several methods of payment for health care,

INTRODUCTION

country can be highly "developed" as far as culture,
education and social structure are concerned, but economically
"poor" and in an early phase of development. On the other
hand, countries can be "rich" and provided with great
economic resources while at the same time being "socially
underdeveloped", i.e. in need of improvement of
educational and social conditions in the broadest sense.
We then should be very careful in stressing that economic
development is only one aspect of overall development.
By the same token, the resources to improve health, which
are the topic of this unit, are not only material and
economic resources, but also those created by and based
on the level of sociocultural strength of a society.

A discussion of health conditions in terms of such quality-
of-life criteria unavoidably must be subjective. For one
reason, the evaluation of health resources depends often on
the point of view and school of thought of the "evaluator."
Furthermore, future development and value of resources
is often not predictable. Nevertheless, it is worthwhile
to examine health problems in terms of their societal
dimensions, because the lack of available resources is
often not the limiting factor in combatting poverty, hunger
and disease so much as the social and political conditions
that prevent these resources from being mobilized and
fairly distributed.

THE ALLOCATION OF HEALTH RESOURCES

Below are two apparently contradictory arguments concerning a global assessment of world resources:

(1)   Based on forward projections of present statistics (demographic data in relation to the rapid depletion of resources including food and minerals), the world's overriding problem is that rapid population growth will outrun any possible **benefits** achieved through the development of resources.

(2)   More than the so-called population explosion, the fact that 25 percent of the world's population consumes more than 85 percent of the world's non-renewable resources accounts for a present day catastrophe which intensifies the degree to which human beings are suffering from substandard living conditions including hunger and disease.

Preassessment

at is your tentative assessment of the global resources
ply? Does it more nearly match the first or second
w? Jot down your thoughts at this point as a preassessing
rcise you will probably want to refer back to later.

If you sided with the first position, you probably looked at the future in terms of the total population our resources will have to serve.   Even if population growth is slowed to the extent it maintains the present growth rate (rather than increasing geometrically, as predicted), our population growth rate is still expected to reach the point where the supply of resources is not sufficient to meet the needs.

If you adopted the second position, you probably were looking at conditions more in terms of the present.   Today there is vast maldistribution of existing resources and resource consumption which could be altered through careful planning and decision-making.

Neither view can be called "right" or "wrong."   The first view was put forth by a multinational group of scientists (the "Club of Rome") in Limits to Growth.   The second view is held by a number of development forecasters in Latin America in the work entitled Catastrophe Or New Society. Certainly, the steady increase of the cost of manufactured and industrial goods mainly produced by the "developed" and "industrialized" countries, and the unpredictable fluc- tuation in the prices of raw materials (generally the principal source of income of the "developing" countries) makes planning and predicting a hazardous task.   There also have been important developments, such as industrialization in previously agricultural mono-culture supported economics (Brazil) and the plant genetics-based "green revolution" in food production (India).   Nevertheless, the great gains made by the discovery of high yield crops have been largely counterbalanced by the increase in the price of oil based fertilizers needed to sustain these crops.   Furthermore, it is clearly the case that much of the world's population is suffering in abject poverty and disease due to malapportione resources.

Is our supply of resources ample enough to "go around?"   Is it possible to bring about the development of improved "human

rvices" and health in poor countries through foreign aid
ograms or through the application of technology? Would
.elp" of some description even be a desirable goal for one
.tion to have in relation to another?

.y, you might ask, does the affluent world participate in the
:velopment of less favored countries? Undoubtedly, altruism --
:sisting the poor in a charitable way -- is one reason.
.king friends (political reasons) and creating more prosperous
.rkets for industrialized societies (economic reasons) are
.hers. As a matter of fact, in most cases these main motives
.nnot be separated and most international development programs
'e based on all three forming the motivating rationale to
varying degree.

THE CONCEPT OF DEVELOPMENT

.ring the past two to three decades, we have witnessed a
.markable change in the approach to international develop-
nt programs. Still influenced by the colonial era, the
nor nations initially insisted on controlling the decision-
.king process in relation to programs in the developing
•rld financed by "foreign aid" and aiming at the improvements
' the quality of life, including health. More often than
•t, this resulted in the transfer of a technology applied
.th some success in the developed world and inappropriate
• the entirely different needs of "backward" societies.
.ny of these developing countries had been colonies and
:re served by whatever health care systems were set up during
•lonial times based on the pattern of the metropolitan
•untry. With the help of foreign assistance programs, the
.wly liberated countries then simply continued or even
panded these systems. Many of these programs were unsuitable
•r the cultural, social, economic, and often special environ-
ntal and epidemiologic health needs of the developing
.untries. The remnants of traditional health care practices,
'ten very useful particularly at the primary care level, were
.t aside and western methodology introduced. Because of
gh cost and sophistication, western style services

were available only to the privileged and mostly urban populations.

Increased nationalism and self-assertion in the developing countries have begun to destroy the vestiges of colonialism. Newly emerging nations are assuming the decision-making activities themselves, even when they operate with foreign or international funds. In spite of this social and political development, improvements and change in the health care programs have not always resulted, in part because the educated classes of both the previously colonized and noncolonized countries had adopted Western values and beliefs. Their leading physicians who dominated the health establishment had been trained in either Europe or the U.S. and had learned to strive towards the priorities of scientific and highly specialized curative medicine rather than preventive medicine and primary care. As a consequence, you will find in most of the developing countries that health services imitate Western models, based in sophisticated hospitals with imported expensive equipment and staffed by personnel trained, often **overtrained, according to the international standards.**

For the mostly urban elites who usually wield the political power, this pattern is quite acceptable. If, however, you venture into the rural areas as well as into the rapidly increasing urban and peri-urban slums, ghettos, bidonvilles, barrios, favelas (or whatever the poverty stricken sections are called), you will find that health services are not available to any considerable degree in these areas, even though the official plans for resource allocation will always include as one goal the total coverage of the population. One of the problems is that "Western-type" services are expensive and drain the meager resources of the health budget. Thus, there are not sufficient funds for the creation of health care delivery systems that are oriented toward urban and rural populations; i.e. primary care and preventive programs.

Below are several examples of population groups in developed and developing countries. Please complete the table by describing the level of affluence you think each group would have and by assessing the health services available to it.

HEALTH SERVICES BY DISTRIBUTION OF RESOURCES

National Level of Affluence	Population Group	Economic Status (high or low)	Provision of Health Services (well or poorly served)
Affluent	Upper class suburb of Paris		
Affluent	Migrant workers in rural California		
Poor	University faculty, Ibadan, Nigeria		
Poor	Squatters in "favelas" (slums of Rio de Janeiro)		

I/4, p. 9

Suggested Responses:

HEALTH SERVICES BY DISTRIBUTION OF RESOURCES

National level of Affluence	Population Group	Economic Status (high or low)	Provision of Health Services (weak or poorly served)
Affluent	Upper class suburb of Paris	*high*	*well served*
Affluent	Migrant workers in rural California	*low*	*poorly served*
Poor	University faculty, Ibadan, Nigeria	*high*	*well served*
Poor	Squatters in "favelas" (slums of Rio de Janeiro)	*low*	*poorly served*

The table is intended to illustrate that poor groups in rich countries can fit the poor country pattern in terms of access to health services just as the elite groups in poor countries often can get very good health care. Other examples of poorly served populations in an affluent country such as the United States are some Indians on reservations, eskimos, "inner city ghetto" populations, and rural groups (e.g. Appalachia, the

ssissippi delta, Southwest Texas, Vermont). In poor
untries populations which probably have access to good
alth care include large landholding families, senior
vernment officials and politicians, diplomats, local
presentatives of international commercial and industrial
ganizations, and professionals, both foreign and domestic.

general, affluence is associated with the political and
cial elite and with access to Western style health services.
rthermore, groups of greater and lesser affluence can be
und in the same country, as well as health systems which
e characterized by the presence or absence of some social
glect. Thus, social inequity, malnutrition, high infant
rtality, poor housing, and the other signs of a poor
andard of living exist among some groups of people in all
untries.

TECHNOLOGICAL DEVELOPMENT

Development, in terms of the quality of life, cannot be
obtained by a simple transfer of technologies from the
industrialized populations enjoying a relatively high
standard of living to the less fortunate population groups
both in the U.S. and abroad. Besides the fact that even
in affluent societies health care delivery and provision
of social services in general have not been an unqualified
success, past experiences have indicated that some technologies and attitudes simply "transferred" have been inappropriate
or even detrimental. Both health problems and the available
resources differ markedly within a country and certainly
between countries. Development encompasses a multiple of
changes. Attempts to achieve development must be concerned
with the individual wishes of each societal group involved.
Decision-makers of these societal groups must be the ones
to determine the "optimal speed" and "provisional cost" of
the changes (See Goulet reference noted on I/4, p. 43).

The ultimate decision of how a country is to use its own
resources and how it will request resources from potential
donor countries and organizations must be left with that
recipient country. In many instances a developing nation will
need assistance in the process of arriving at such decisions.
If at all possible, such assistance is provided by otherwise
uninvolved organizations; for instance, in the health field,
by the World Health Organization. Obviously, where technical
and/or financial assistance is involved in the development
process, the "donor societies" have the right and responsibility to take part in the decision-making and planning
activities, but the decision-making cannot be left to them
alone.

e characteristic role of the United States in the develop-
nt of poor countries has been much debated in recent years,
d assessed this way:

n our prescription for the improvement of other countries,
 have a little-recognized tendency to advocate what exists
 the United States with no critical view as to its appropri-
eness to the situation or stage of development of other
untries." -- John Kenneth Galbraith

thin its global role of assistance, the United States
obably should try to avoid the kind of pitfall that Galbraith
rceives. Technology transfer and resource allocation must
come a truly cooperative venture of donor, recipient, and
eutral" organizations, countries and individuals, recognizing
at there are no universal solutions and methods which apply
 all, and that each health care delivery system has to be
aped taking into consideration the multiple social factors
 each population group and country. The role of the experts
en does not consists of attempts to simply transfer techno-
gies, proven or unproven in their own countries, but of
sistance in identifying, analyzing and evaluating problems
d their solutions.

DEVELOPMENT OF PREVENTIVE, CURATIVE, AND REHABILITATIVE SERVICES

In many parts of the world certain diseases and health problems are so prevalent as to constitute a serious hindrance to development. In some cases these diseases could be prevented from occurring; in others, the diseases are curable; and in some instances diseases are susceptible to rehabilitative treatment, or a combination of the three. Thus, depending on the problem, health resources may be more profitably allocated for one type of service than another. Let us take as an example, Poliomyelitis: it is fully preventable (vaccination), essentially not curable when contracted, and not susceptible to full rehabilitation of function. Therefore, the development of an effective vaccination program would constitute the wisest allocation of resources for health services among those countries in which poliomyelitis is a health problem.

Exercise

By way of an exercise in considering diseases in terms of an efficient allocation of health resources for health services, complete Table 1 on the next page, as we have done for poliomyelitis. Put a (+) in Column A if you think that a condition is fully preventable; a (+ -) if partially preventable; and a (-) if the condition cannot be treated with that form of health service. Do the same in Columns B (curable condition) and C (suceptible to rehabilitation).

TABLE 1

DISEASE TREATMENT THROUGH THREE TYPES OF HEALTH SERVICE

	A	B	C
	Preventable	Curable	Susceptible to Rehabilitation
Poliomyelitis	+	−	+ −
Smallpox			(n/a)
Measles			(n/a)
Diarrhea			(n/a)
Schistosomiasis			
Tetanus			
Ancylostomiasis			
Chagas' disease (South American Trypanosomiasis)			
Sleeping sickness (African Trypanosomiasis)			
Tuberculosis			
Onchocerciasis			
Amebiasis			
Cholera			(n/a)
Gonorrhea			
Syphilis			
Pneumonia by Mycoplasma			(n/a)
Malnutrition			
Population Growth			
Coronary Heart Disease			
Cancer			
Hypertension			
Leukemia			
Rheumatoid Arthritis			
Alcoholism			

Suggested Responses: *Although you may feel some are debatabl*
the following judgements about each of the listed diseases
are suggested.

TABLE 1

	A	B	C
	Preventable	Curable	Susceptible to Rehabilitation
Poliomyelitis	+ -	+ -	+ -
Smallpox	+	-	(n/a)
Measles	+	-	(n/a)
Diarrhea	+ -	+ -	(n/a)
Schistosomiasis	+	-	-
Tetanus	+	+ -	(n/a)
Ancylostomiasis	+	+	-
Chagas' disease (South American Trypanosomiasis)	-	+ -	-
Sleeping sickness (African Trypanosomiasis)	+ -	+	-
Tuberculosis	+ -	+	+ -
Onchocerciasis	+ -	-	-
Amebiasis	+ -	+	-
Cholera	+ -	+	(n/a)
Gonorrhea	+ -	+	+
Syphilis	+ -	+	+
Pneumonia by Mycoplasma	-	-	(n/a)
Malnutrition	+	+	+
Population Growth	+	-	-
Coronary Heart Disease	+ -	+ -	+ -
Cancer	-	+ -	+ -
Hypertension	-	+ -	+ -
Leukemia	-	-	-
Rheumatoid Arthritis	-	-	+ -
Alcoholism	-	-	+ -

Conceivably, one might measure the quality of care in terms
of identified diseases -- unnecessary (preventable) diseases,

seases that cause unnecessary or untimely deaths (are
sceptible to curative care), and/or diseases that cause
necessary disability (are susceptible to rehabilitative
asures). However, whether it be to assess the quality
care or to plan for the allocation of health resources
:hin a given society, the strategy ought to involve the
e following steps:

Determine the most important health problems.

Classify these problems as susceptible to preventive
and/or curative and/or rehabilitative measures.

Calculate the cost of such measures applied effectively.

Determine the priorities for intervention.

en it comes to the allocation of resources, the same
oblem plagues all societies from the most affluent to
e least developed: How much effort should be expended
curative, preventive and rehabilitative services?
obably you have realized that the disease pattern in the
:luent and the developing societies varies greatly.*

:VENTION

.le curative followed by rehabilitative measures are
licated for most of the diseases of populations with a
;h standard of living, vast numbers of people throughout
e world lack even the simplest measures of health care.
·y suffer and are dying from preventable conditions
;ociated with poor housing and sanitation, malnutrition,
·asitic, and infectious diseases aggravated by overpopula-
·n. Under these conditions, a program skewed toward pre-
1tive methods is indicated. The recent singular success

---

* A fuller discussion of these disease patterns is
sented in Unit I/2, "Worldwide Patterns of Disease."

of the worldwide smallpox eradication program is an example
of such a successful approach.

In contrast, with malaria we have used insect control for many
years as the main preventive measure and have made great advances, but have encountered social and economic conditions
which precluded the use of such means. In addition to vector
control, a safe and effective vaccine is needed. Here is one
area in which the scientific establishment of the affluent
societies could assist the developing world with a technologica
achievement and transfer.

CURE

There is no clear cut difference between preventive and curative measures. Often the treatment and ultimate cure of a
disease is an effective preventive measure, as for instance
in tuberculosis, where chemotherapy eliminates the danger
of the spread of the tubercle bacilli, making careful case
finding and treatment of the infected individuals the most
effective preventive measure fot the population-at-large.
That naturally does not mean that the largely effective BCG
vaccination and general improvement of sanitary conditions
should be neglected.

Another example in which preventive and curative measures have
to be combined is hookworm disease (ancylostomiasis), probably
the most widespread and debilitating parasitic disease on
earth. It is curable without too much difficulty, but the
cured individual usually is reinfected in his home environment
because simple preventive behavior such as the use of latrines
is not followed. Building of latrines needed for the prevention of a number diseases as well as sanitary education of the
people, would go a long way toward the improvement of health.
Clean water supply and food preservation are other important
measures.

REHABILITATION

For individuals who are either cured or partially cured with
a remaining functional capability there is a need for

:habilitative services. To make life enjoyable and to
.intain them as productive members of society, physical and
.otional rehabilitation should be an important function of
.e health care provider in addition to curative and preven-
.ve activities.

. the final analysis, the greatest difficulty in implementing
.is triple role as provider of preventive, curative and
:habilitative care, lies in the overwhelming prestige of
.e healer of dysfunction and suffering. The relief of pain
.d disability by opening three abscesses is vastly more
.mired and appreciated than the vaccination of the whole
.llage against smallpox, measles, tuberculosis, tetanus,
.d diphtheria. One must be realistic and recognize that in
.cing the excess of illness throughout the developing world,
.e most urgent task may be that of convincing the health
.re providers to give less emphasis to curative activities.
.evention and rehabilitation should be held at the same
.iority level as curative services. Frequently, attempts
. emphasize preventive and rehabilitative services are made
.re difficult because the consumers will not accept preventive
.ograms, including family planning, without simultaneous
.ovision of curative services.

.vertheless, the cost of health care delivery has become an
.tolerable burden, even for the affluent societies. For
.e developing countries, which often have to start from
.ratch in the formation of all their social institutions,
. is even more critical that the most effective services are
.eated and maintained at the lowest cost and greatest
.ficiency possible.

THE USE OF HUMAN RESOURCES

. the center of the planning for better health care delivery
. the question of health manpower. Although it is generally
.cepted that a "health team" is well suited to manage health
.re at the national, community, and even family level, the
.mposition of that team is still a matter of discussion.
.at should it include in the way of physicians? Nurse
.actitioners? Auxiliary health workers? Medical assistants?

I/4, p. 19

Nurse-midwives? physician extenders? feldshers? barefoot
doctors? and so forth.

COMPOSITION

There is a great variety of health workers from which to draw
a health team. There is a reasonable consensus that the
physician, traditionally the sole or at least the usual
responsible provider of care, must now share that responsibility
with other health professionals. There is rapid population
growth and increasing demand for health services
larly in the developing countries, aggravated by the fact
that many have lost health coverage provided by their previous
colonial masters. As a result, much of the health care is
given today by other health professionals. This is probably
desirable because again, cultural, social, economic, demographic, and other locally determined influences make flexi-
bility and adaptability absolutely necessary. No pattern
can be universal. It is vitally important, however, that
the various members of this team have clearly identifiable
roles and tasks. Often, if available, physicians will assume
the role of leadership, but in many instances, at the local
level, the non-physician health care providers must be given
full responsibilities. It also must not be forgotten that
certainly the majority of people throughout the world do not
have contact with a health care system as we conceive it,
based on "Western" medicine and culture. They seek and
receive help from a large array of healers, often called
"traditional providers" with names like "curanderos" (South
America); "Ayurvedics" (India, Nepal); "bomos" (Malaysia);
"herbateros" (South America); "shamans" (Siberia); "acupunc-
turists" (China); "macumbeiros" (Brazil); "mufumus", "babalawos
"onisheguns" (Africa); "medicine men" and "sages femmes --
wise women" (many societies) and numerous others. And even
in the affluent countries, where Western medicine is dominant,
the role of faith healers, chiropractic practitioners and
other providers outside the "regular health system" is a
very important one. Under no circumstances should one under-
estimate the contribution made by these traditional healers.

ulturally and socially they are often much nearer to the
consumer of their services and more atuned to their emotional
needs and societal constraints. In some instances, but not
often enough, it has been demonstrated that an integration
or at least partial integration of the traditional healers
and the Western health care providers can be very effective
in both raising the quality of care and increasing the
quantity of available manpower. China seems to have succeeded
in combining training for practice in traditional and western
medicine. Just one other example is the training of traditional "partera" (village midwife) in Latin America in
aseptic techniques, resulting in a sharp reduction of tetanus.

Since the problem of an insufficient number of health care
providers will be with us for a long time, we should be
thinking of ways to minimize the shortage or otherwise trying
to meet health service needs. There are several things
which have a bearing on manpower supply. For example, an
increased emphasis should be placed on public health education
leading to the lay person's involvement in his own care,
both preventive and curative. There is a great deal individuals
can do for themselves to lower the ever increasing cost of
health care and to relieve the problems of under supply, as
well as maldistribution of health manpower.

URBAN AND RURAL DISTRIBUTION

Another problem of resource allocation concerns the distribution of services to urban and rural areas. It is often
stated that the most serious problem in the developing
world is the neglect of rural areas , in terms of both
health and social services. In most rural areas a good deal
of the responsibility for care must be assumed by non-physic ian
health workers (traditional healers and paramedical personnel).

Despite the concern for rural health care, one could argue that the major health and social problems in the coming decades will be in the underprivileged urban centers. How is this argument supported by Figure 1, which demonstrates real and projected population increases in major cities between 1950 and 2000?

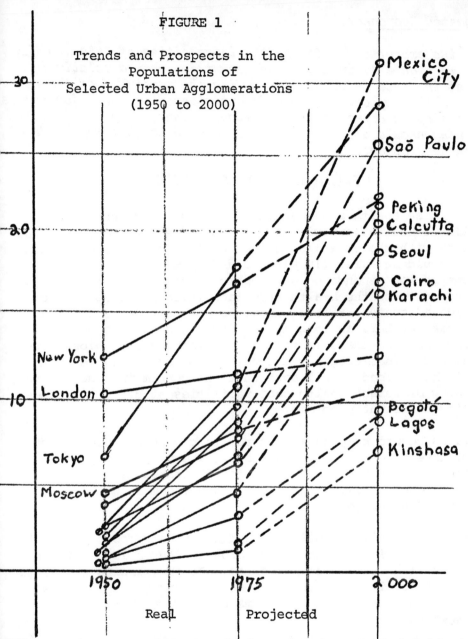

FIGURE 1

Trends and Prospects in the
Populations of
Selected Urban Agglomerations
(1950 to 2000)

Mexico City
Saõ Paulo
Peking
Calcutta
Seoul
Cairo
Karachi
New York
London
Bogotá
Lagos
Kinshasa
Tokyo
Moscow

30

20

10

1950   1975   2000

Real   Projected

SOURCE: Working Paper #58, Population Division, United Nations
(November 21, 1975).

Suggested Responses:

With the exception of Tokyo, the large cities of 1950 (to the left in Figure 1) in developed countries show a relatively modest increase in population during the remainder of the century, while explosive growth is anticipated in the major cities of developing countries (right side). Thus, long range health planning should allow for services geared to this magnitude of urban development.

HEALTH CARE ORGANIZATION

To minimize health and planning problems and to employ the available health manpower in the most effective way, regionalization with the establishment of different levels of health care should be carefully planned and implemented. The size of one region depends on geographic factors and principally on the capacity of the health care facilities and manpower to provide adequate service. It would not make sense to give arbitrary numbers as long as the decisions have to be made on the basis of these factors and preferably some biostatistical and epidemiological evaluations or even surveys. It should be avoided at all cost that the consumers "shop around," choosing different health care facilities at different times and for different problems.

It makes record keeping and therewith continuous and effective preventive care all but impossible. The very widespread practice of entering the system for the first time through the emergency services for non-emergency complaints should be strongly discouraged.

Orderly, effective, continuous and relatively economic health care is probably best provided through a three level system. Figure 2 illustrates such a system. As an exercise in identifying various levels within the health care system, please label the diagram using the terms in the box at the top of the next page.

USE EACH OF THESE GIVEN TERMS TO LABEL FIGURE 2:

(1) PRIMARY CARE   (consumer entry point into health care
                         system)
(2) SECONDARY CARE   (point of referral for hospital care)
(3) TERTIARY CARE   (central point for sophisticated health
                         services offered on a regional basis)

(4) 65-80% of patients are treated at this level
(5) 5-10% of patients are treated at this level
(6) 15-25% of patients are treated at this level
(7) Community hospital (CH)
(8) Regional hospital
(9) Health post (HP)

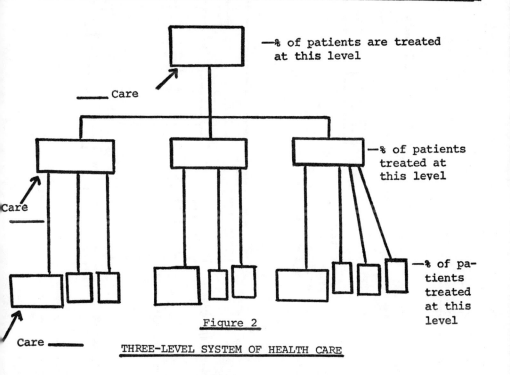

Figure 2

THREE-LEVEL SYSTEM OF HEALTH CARE

I/4, p. 25

Suggested Response:

Figure 2

THREE-LEVEL SYSTEM OF HEALTH CARE

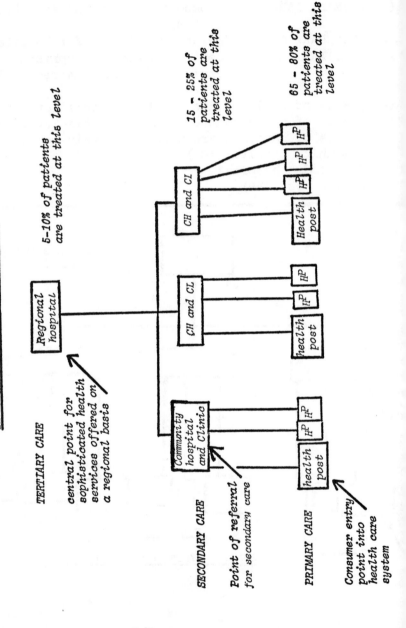

TERTIARY CARE

*central point for
sophisticated health
services offered on
a regional basis*

5-10% of patients
are treated at this level

SECONDARY CARE

*Point of referral
for secondary care*

PRIMARY CARE

*Consumer entry
point into
health care
system*

15 - 25% of
patients are
treated at this
level

65 - 80% of
patients are
treated at this
level

et's look more closely at these three levels of health care.

PRIMARY CARE

Primary care is defined as first contact with continuous follow-up. It should be given in the community, preferably as ambulatory services in health posts without inpatient facilities. Depending on available health manpower, this can be done by physicians, obviously generalists; but in a more economical program paramedical and auxiliary personnel, specially trained for primary care, are perfectly capable of performing at this level. This population should receive general health education in these posts and should learn to accept them as the site for continuous preventive and, if necessary, curative care and as the point of entry into the health care system. Home care and home visits to incapacitated, elderly and otherwise house-bound patients should be one of the responsibilities of these health posts. To give one example: distribution of drugs and supervision of drug taking in tuberculosis, which is the decisive activity in the control of this disease, should be done at the health post level in a much more effective way than in the impersonal, relatively inaccessible large hospital clinic. In general, the health post could provide care in a much more personalized, continuous and humane fashion. Experiences in many programs have shown that between 65% and 80% of all first contacts can be taken care of at this level at a very low cost (about 1/15 to 1/20 of the "per diem" cost in a tertiary hospital).

SECONDARY CARE

Only those patients who need additional diagnostic methods, sophisticated therapy, the expertise of a physician and/or hospitalization, have to be referred from the primary care health post. Usually, about 20% of the first contacts and never more than 35% fall into that category.

Fifteen to 25% will have their health problem dealth with at the secondary health care level which consists of ambulatory

care and inpatient services with general diagnostic and
therapeutic facilities and staffed by generalists, both
physicians and paramedical personnel. Very often, existing
community hospitals can be adapted and the "per diem" cost
can be kept consistently at less than half the cost of the
tertiary hospital.

TERTIARY CARE

Only five to ten percent need care at the tertiary level,
a hospital staffed by specialists and equipped with the
most modern and advanced diagnostic and therapeutic tools.
Its "per diem" cost is rapidly rising everywhere (in the
U.S. it has reached approximately U.S. $200.00). Not every
tertiary regional hospital should have extremely expensive
services like open-heart surgery, renal transplantation
and dialysis facilities, cobalt therapy units and so forth.
Referrals to those services, often localized in a university
connected hospital with renowned faculty members, will be
made from other parts of the country and even other countries.

It must be stressed that teaching and training activities
as well as research have to be conducted at all levels to
guarantee future health manpower, some with the ability to
provide primary and others specialized care.

Finally, it must be said emphatically that in most cases this
briefly described health care system cannot be created at
once. It represents something similar to "a final solution."
The officials responsible to allocate resources, however,
should keep in mind that with the gradual implementation of
such a system, cost-effectiveness can be significantly
improved.

FINANCING HEALTH SERVICES AND REIMBURSING PHYSICIANS

Economic and political factors determine to a large degree
the health personnel, facilities and system in which they
are utilized. Different countries have developed and adopted

:ious systems of payment for health care. As a matter
fact, health care in many countries including the
;. is financed not by one uniform system but by a mixture
programs, some based on fee-for-service, others private
surance, and still others, government support.*

alth economists have discussed at great length whether
alth care should be financed and organized through the
:ket or by government. Obviously the political philosophy
each government ultimately determines the fate of all
:vices given to the population. If the government is
dicated to the egalitarian approach, then health care is
so organized in an egalitarian way, that is, equal care
: everyone according to need and regardless of financial
ans and social status. It is fair to say that, at least
eoretically, all political systems today recognize health
:e as a right for all citizens, and strive to provide
alitarian care with more or less success.

)ER FORMS OF MEDICAL PRACTICE

der the older forms of medical practice in the Western
:ld in which individual physicians and individual patients
intained a direct and private relationship between provider
1 consumer, or seller and buyer, it was often said that
:ients of limited financial means were unable to obtain
ality care, that physicians chose more remunerative special-
es rather than those which were badly needed, including
blic health and preventive medicine, and that physicians
so elected to practice in the more affluent cities rather
an in the countryside. In more extreme cases, physicians
:e accused of performing more rewarding, unnecessary services
:her than the necessary, beneficial but unchallenging
es. All this created a dual value system in medical care.

_____

ne organizational and economic aspects of health care
stems will be discussed in greater detail in Category V.
this introductory unit, only an overview is given.

A citation from antiquity, "The Laws" by Plato, indicates that
this duality in the physician's role is an old problem:

> "And did you ever observe that there are two classes
> of patients in states, slaves and freemen; and the
> slave doctors run about and cure the slaves, or
> wait for them in the dispensaries—practitioners
> of this sort never talk to their patients individ-
> ually, or let them talk about their own individual
> complaints? The slave-doctor prescribes what mere
> experience suggests, as if he had exact knowledge;
> and when he has given his orders, like a tyrant,
> he rushes off with equal assurance to some other
> servant who is ill; and so he relieves the master
> of the house of the care of his invalid slaves.
> But the other doctor, who is a freeman, attends
> and practices upon freemen; and he carries his
> enquiries far back, and goes into the nature of
> the disorder; he enters into discourse with the
> patient and with his friends, and is at once getting
> information from the sick man, and also instructing
> him as far as he is able, and he will not prescribe
> for him until he has first convinced him; at last,
> when he brought the patient more and more under his
> persuasive influences and set him on the road to
> health, he attempts to effect a cure. Now which
> is the better way of proceeding in a physician
> and in a trainer?"

In most societies, such a difference between the availability and quality of health care for those who are able
to purchase it themselves and those who have to rely on
others including the government to pay for it, persists
to-date. Even the socialist countries, who proclaim their
dedication to an egalitarian society, have not yet reached
the goal of providing uniform health services to the
whole population.

erywhere, however, pressure is being exerted to improve
e organization and financing of medical care through
blic action. In many instances, workers, farmers and
en the unemployed, the aged and other previously under-
ivileged groups have gained increased political power
d have used it to demand, among other social benefits
proved health care. Sometimes, authoritarian governments
ve also given extended medical services to the oppressed
pulations in order to gain approval of the otherwise
stile lower classes. Two forms of overall organizations
ve been most widely used: National Health Insurance and
tional Health Services. Even though they are often
nfused, they are really quite distinct.

tional Health Insurance schemes are widely employed in
st European countries and other affluent countries such
Australia, for example, and in the United States in a some-
at unusual and, one might say, incomplete form.

tional Health Services are still relatively rare. The
viet Union and other Eastern European countries have delivered
alth services under that system for several decades, as
ve Great Britain and the People's Republic of China.
at differs fundamentally in these two systems is the
thod of financing. Under National Health Insurance
ployers and/or employees, through tax levies, pay for
e insurance and, consequently, only the employees, in
st instances with their dependents, are covered and have
e right to more or less extensive medical care. Under
tional Health Services all care is funded by the national
easury and, therefore, every citizen, and often even every
sident, is fully covered.

w are the actual medical bills paid? How is the doctor
other health provider paid? Under all coverage systems
ere are several possible ways of paying doctors and other
alth service providers.

METHODS OF REIMBURSING PHYSICIANS

<u>Fee-For-Service</u>: Under the fee-for-service scheme, each health-related procedure, either curative, preventive or rehabilitative, is paid for separately. This can be done either directly by an insurance company, government agency or sick fund, or by the consumer who is then reimbursed by one of them, usually referred to as "third party." This fee-for-service system, particularly the one in which the consumer pays the provider, resembles most the traditional type of medical practice, based on a very personal doctor-patient relationship and free choice of the provider. Nevertheless, it also presents some problems: there is a tendency to employ **more expensive procedures and** in general to overtreat and overattend patients; surgery might be used instead of **some more conservative medical treatment, injections instead of orally administered drugs, and prolonged hospitalization instead of out-patient care.**

<u>Capitation</u>: Under the system of capitation, each provider has a list of patients regularly assigned to him and he is supposed to take care of all of their health-related needs. He receives a fixed annual payment for each of his patients, even for those who never seek his help. On the other hand, he also collects only the regular fee for a patient who needs and demands unusual attention. Since this system covers only the relationship between one provider and the consumer, in most countries using the capitation system (among them Italy, Spain, the Netherlands), it only covers the family physician. Referrals to specialists and other health care facilities must be taken care of separately. While this system clearly does not favor excessive care and unnecessary procedures, it tends to err in the opposite direction. Time consuming patients might be easily referred a; in general, there is little incentive for very careful and frequent attention to the patient.

<u>Salaries</u>: Salaries are paid to providers according to time spent and usually according to their rank. The payment is

de directly by the "third party" and is in no way
influenced by the provider-consumer relationship. This
system is therefore the least favored by the traditional
professional associations and organizations. It is said
to foster hasty care, unnecessary referrals, excessive
control of the government or other "third party" bureaucracy
and destruction of the doctor-patient relationship, particularly since in this system there is only a limited choice
of providers, if any. On the other hand, in addition to
economical care the defenders of salaried health care cite
as advantages non-mercenary attitudes, less bookkeeping for the
provider, better relationships between the various health professionals, and continuity and safety for the consumer in times
of catastrophic illness.

One of the reasons why you may find it so difficult to
evaluate global health progress, is that invariably difficult plans are being tried and different levels of progress
coexist in every society, and that therefore the relative
benefits and shortcomings cannot be measured separately with
any degree of exactness and confidence. For example, in
terms of the various methods for reimbursement, the
physicians in Britain treat patients both under the National
Health Service and privately. Patients eligible for
free care, even in the Socialist countries, may elect
private care because they feel that they might obtain earlier
appointments, longer attention and generally better care, and
indeed as long as the mixture of private and public care
and payments persist, that might be true in most cases.

A UNIT REVIEW

While the "resources to improve health" are often material and economic in nature, they also are dependent on the level of sociocultural strength of a society. The purpose of this unit has been to look broadly at the development of health resources from the standpoint of "social medicine."

The following statements are intended to help you summarize and review some of the major points. Please check all of the items that help to explain each summary statement.

1. Scarcity of resources. Resources are scarce. There are not enough to go around and the resource supply is becoming increasingly dear.

___(a) More than three fourths of the world's resources are being consumed by only one fourth of its population.

___(b) Sophisticated secondary and tertiary care facilities provide elitist groups in even some of the poorest countries with excellent curative care

___(c) Technological developments can rapidly render obsolete long range projection based on present rates at which supplies and materials are being consumed.

___(d) Global population growth rates are continuing to increase.

The sociocultural backdrop for development.

espite having the know-how to provide efficient and effective
alth service systems, many countries have <u>not</u> developed
eir health resources wisely.

_(a) Most developing countries emulate western health
    service systems, based in sophisticated hospitals
    with imported expensive equipment and overtrained
    personnel

_(b) Those few countries which focus most of their health
    resources on the development of primary care services
    actually are helping to meet 60 - 85% of the health
    needs.

_(c) Historically, foreign aid and technology experts have
    tended to be accompanied by prescriptions for develop-
    ment efforts to proceed along the lines of affluent
    country development, rather than assistance in helping
    the developing country to identify, analyze and
    evaluate problems and solutions.

Suggested Responses:

1. *a,b,d*

2. *a,e*

3. Development of preventive, curative and rehabilitative services. How much effort should be expended on each kind of service? This is often difficult to determine.

___(a) There is often no clear difference between prevention and cure. Tuberculosis can be combatted either through chemotherapy (which eliminates the danger of spreading the disease) or by vaccinating the population at large and improving general sanitary conditions.

___(b) The healer of dysfunction and suffering is accorded more respect everywhere than is the health worker who successfully but unceremonially vaccinates a group of people against smallpox.

___(c) The cost of health service is so high that even affluent countries are finding it advantageous to stress disease prevention rather than long-term curative and rehabilitative services.

<u>Development of Human Resources.</u> In the center of health
planning efforts is the question of health manpower.
Although the "health team" is an accepted concept,
its composition is still a matter of discussion.

_(a) In most countries the physician is the sole provider
    of care.

_(b) The majority of countries throughout the world make
    use of "traditional providers" such as medicine men
    and sages femmes (wise women) or providers outside
    the regular health system (e.g. faith healers,
    chiropractors).

_(c) In some areas of the world (China and Latin America),
    efforts have successfully been made to combine the
    training for and practice in traditional and western
    medicine, as with the village midwife.

3. *a, b, c*
4. *b, c*

B. Economic and political factors determine to a large degree the health personnel, facilities and system in which they are utilized. Especially in terms of physician reimbursement, different countries have developed and adopted various systems of payment for health care. In the space below, name and briefly **explain** three methods of physician compensation.

(1) _____

_____

_____

(2) _____

_____

_____

(3) _____

_____

_____

. Which of these reimbursement methods do you think is least
ell suited to the development of an efficient health service
ystem in a poor country? Why?

Suggested Responses:

B. *You should have included the three listed below (in any order). Your explanations should have approximated the following:*

    (1) fee-for-service -- each health-related procedure is paid for separately.

    (2) Capitation -- a fixed amount is paid on the basis of a list of regularly assigned patients for whom the provider renders health service.

    (3) Salary -- a sum is paid to the provider according to rank and time spent on health services.

C. *The fee-for-service method of payment is least suited to the development of a health service system in a poor country. This is because the physician under the fee system must perform a particular usually curative procedure in order to be reimbursed whereas under a capitation or a salaried system preventive health measures are reimbursed as fully as curative efforts. This is important, especially since national health insurance and health service programs have removed the financial constraints which previously forced a patient to curtail consumption of curative services when they exceeded his ability to pay.*

You should discuss questions and points of interest with your instructor. In addition, you might consult some of the references listed **below for further information.**

REFERENCES

ckington, F. *World Health*. Churchill Livingstone
nburgh, London and New York, 1975.
   An overview of the principal world health problems,
   with special elaboration of the history of international
   cooperation and the activities and problems of WHO.

ant, J. *Health and the Development World*. Cornell
versity Press, Ithaca and London, 1969.
   A fundamental analysis of the health status of the
   world's poor, based on broad statistics as well as
   on the author's extensive experience.

ill, K.M. *The Untapped Resource*. Orbis Books, New York,
71.
   This book poses the challenge to the US to use its
   wealth and power to fight ill health throughout the
   world. The author believes that this is "an untapped
   resource of contemporary international diplomacy."

, J. *Medicine in Three Societies*. American Elsevier
lishing Co., Inc. New York, 1970.
   A comparison of medical care in the USSR, USA and UK

let, D. *The Cruel Choice, A New Concept in the Theory of
velopment*. Atheneum, New York, 1971.
   An unconventional and critical evaluation of development
   policies, stressing the moral and ethical implications of
   aid and technology transfer, decided and implemented by
   a modernizing elite rather than by the affected people.

rera, O., Scolnik, H.D., Chichilnisky, G., Gallopin, G.C.,
doy, J.E., Mosovich, D., Oteiza, E., de Romero Brest, G.L.,
rez, C.E., and Talavera, L. *Catastrophe or New Society?
Latin American World Model*. International Development
earch Center, Ottawa, 1976.

Kaplan, M. "Risks and Rewards," World Health. The Magazine of the WHO, June 1976, p. 12.
Report of a special round table discussion on biomedical research organized by WHO's Office of Research Promotion and Development.

Knowles, J.H. "The Struggle to Stay Healthy," TIME, August 9, 1976, p. 60.
Analysis of the history and philosophy of development of better health care.

Meadows, D.H., Meadows, D.L., Randers, J., Behrens, Wm. W. 3rd. Limits to Growth: a Report on the Club of Rome's Project on the Predicament of Mankind. 2nd edition, Universe Books, Inc., New York, 1974.
A projection of the future problems of mankind, based on careful and systematic analysis of resources, population growth and related factors.

Myrdal, G. Asian Drama. Inquiry Into the Poverty of Nations. Pantheon, New York, 1968.
An extensive (3 volumes) and detailed presentation of the social problems, including health, facing the developing countries, using Southeast Asia as the source for many examples, but valid for most of the developing world.

Orihuela, L.A. "Where the Streetlamps Stop," World Health, the Magazine of the World Health Organization, May 1976, p. 23.
A description of the health and other social problems of the populations of the major metropoles of the world.

Rutstein, D.D., Berenberg, W., Chalmers, T.C., Child, 3rd, C.G., Fishman, A.P., and Perrin, E.B. "Measuring the Quality of Medical Care: A Clinical Method." New England Journal of Medicine 294:582-588 (1976)
An innovative approach to measurement of quality of care, applicable to planning of health care delivery.

rner, F.C. "The Rush to the Cities," in <u>Latin America Science</u>, 2:955 (1976)
   Article on reasons and effects of the rapid migration from rural to urban areas in Latin Americal

rd, B. (Lady Jackson) <u>The Rich Nations and the Poor Nations</u>, W. Norton & Co., New York, 1962.
   A short, concise presentation of the dilemma the world is facing in relation to the widening gap between the affluent and the "developing" countries.

alth. <u>Sector Policy Paper.</u> World Bank, 1975.
   A description of programs and methods which the World Bank plans to use in the health field.

alth by the People. Edited by Kenneth W. Newell, WHO neva, 1975.
   A collection of articles by a multi-national group of health care planners dealing with the specific problems of third world countries.

collection of papers and conferences on "The Professional hool and World Affairs," <u>Internationalizing the U.S. ofessional School Occasional Report No. 9.</u> Education and rld Affairs, New York, 1969.

port of the "Institute on International Medical Education" tended by numerous health manpower experts from many untries. <u>Manpower for the World's Health</u>, edited by . v.Z. Hyde, Association of American Medical Colleges, anston, 1966.

UNIT I/5: INTERNATIONAL COOPERATION IN HEALTH

DIETER KOCH-WESER, M.D., PH.D.

CONTENTS

OBJECTIVES

Whether you are planning for an international health
experience as a student, are certain about career
opportunities in international health, or simply interested
in the way the community of nations handles health problems,
you will find (if you go into the field in any depth at all)
a myriad of organizations involved in international health.
The purpose of this unit is to survey, in a very general
way, international cooperation in organizing and financing
health programs. After completing the unit you should
be able to:

1. Explain why nations and private organizations undertake
international health activities.

2. State three types of organizations involved in international health and describe the particular strengths
and weaknesses of each.

3. State the limitations and opportunities available
to you if you decide to pursue your international
interests overseas.

4. Cite at least two of the major obstacles to international
cooperation in health.

INTRODUCTION

In the "Annual Register of Grant Support" in the United
States (see reference at end of unit), more than a hundred
programs are listed, which are totally or partially devoted
to international health activities. Why? What's "in it"
for them? What do they get out of international health
involvement? Why, for example, did Sweden, the United
States and France spend on non-military foreign aid such
disparate amounts as .72, .25 and .60 percent or the
gross national product? No doubt, there are many reasons.

ter in the unit you will be asked to try to explain why
ere is international cooperation in health matters.
rst, however, consider the following.

1Y COOPERATE IN INTERNATIONAL HEALTH ACTIVITIES?

TRUISM

e of the major reasons for "foreign aid" activities should
 recognized as altruism. The average per capita income of
person living in an underdeveloped country is $280 per
ar, compared with $3,670 for an individual residing in an
dustrialized country. Whether it be guilt or the
manitarian accoutrements of society, there is a "feeling"
 the part of people in affluent societies that there should
 a sharing of wealth, skills, knowledge and health manpower
th those in less affluent countries.

LITICAL AND ECONOMIC STABILITY

e U.S. Census Bureau released a report in September 1976
dicating that three of every four persons on earth in
75 were from underdeveloped country. However, these
ree-fourths of the world's population control only about
e-third of the world's aggregate wealth. Furthermore,
e gap between rich and poor nations is widening. Worldwide
litical stability and security as well as sound economics
pend clearly on the improvement of the standard of living
 the "poor nations." International assistance including
d in the health field, therefore, is not only indicated
r altruistic reasons alone, but for self-preservation
 the affluent societies as well.

re directly, the rapid development of technology of
ansportation and communication has produced a rapidly
rinking world, in which cooperation in many fields,
cluding health, has become mandatory. Furthermore, of all
e so-called assitance programs which have come more and

more under attack in the third world as weapons of
imperialism and even "neo colonial" intentions, those
aimed at improvement of health conditions are the least
open to criticism. In a somewhat paradoxical way, these
apparently apolitical health programs can go far in
creating a favorable and trusting relationship between
countries. (It must be stressed at this point that family
planning activities which often have become the mainstay of
health assistance programs, are not always accepted with
the same apolitical attitude. Family planning activities
must be dealt with in a very special way, paying special
attention to political, cultural, religious, and other
social factors in order to respond to the need for population
control . Since World War II, "foreign aid" to developing
countries has been a way of life in affluent nations
(see Figure 1). It is also widely accepted that only
"non-military foreign aid" should be considered as real
development aid and should be separated administratively
and ideologically from the supply of weapons and other
"military aid."

ADVANCES IN HEALTH CARE TECHNOLOGY AND THE ORGANIZATION OF
SERVICES

From the technical and professional point of view, most
international activities are cooperative rather than
assistance programs, although the economic burden is usually
carried by the affluent countries. Health, health training
and health research do not know national boundaries and
thus the knowledge gained from a discovery in one part of
the world often can be profitably applied in other settings.
For example, many of the technical and scientific advances
in medicine that have occurred in developed countries are
readily adopted for use in less developed countries that
cannot   afford to conduct the extensive research leading
up to the discovery. By the same token, a poor country
cannot make a serious attempt to meet the health care needs
of its people by spending its precious health dollars

1974 NON-MILITARY FOREIGN AID

In Millions of U.S. Dollars

SWEDEN	$401.7
NETH.	$428.8
FRANCE	$1,638.4
NORWAY	$131.4
CANADA	$713.4
BRITAIN	$721.8
W. GERMANY	$1,434.6
U.S.	$3,439.0
JAPAN	$1,126.2

Per Cent of G.N.P.

Country	Per Cent
SWEDEN	.72
NETH.	.62
FRANCE	.60
NORWAY	.57
CANADA	.50
BRITAIN	.38
W. GERMANY	.36
U.S.	.25
JAPAN	.25

Source: O.E.C.D.

I/5, p. 5

according to the same health priorities that apply to a
country such as Canada. In many instances the developing
nations have evolved innovative solutions to their health
care delivery problem.

New approaches to health care have already been implemented
in countries with a great variety of socio-economic systems,
cultural traditions and religious and traditional beliefs.
By cooperating in these innovative health programs,
individuals, institutions and organizations from the affluent
countries can learn a great deal about egalitarian health
care delivery systems, the use of non-physician health care
providers, the acceptance and integration of traditional
and other "non-Western." health care practices, and other ways
of containing the rise of health care cost   In addition,
valuable experience can be gained with preventive and
curative projects, much less available in the affluent
countries, such as those in the fields of nutrition, infectious
and tropical diseases, vaccination campaigns and in general
health problems related to poverty.

WHAT KINDS OF ORGANIZATIONS UNDERTAKE
INTERNATIONAL HEALTH ACTIVITIES

here are many different types of organizations involved in
international health. Some are governmental; others private.
ome have health as their major goal; others have it as only
 small part of a broad-spectrum program. These organizations may conduct bilateral programs (carry out programs
involving two countries only) or maintain a multilateral
genda (decisions are made) jointly by representation from
ore than two countries). For the purposes of discussion,
e will classify these organizations as: bilateral
governmental or non-governmental) and multilateral.

irtually all "affluent" countries parallel the U.S. in that
hey have government agencies, private non-profit and profit
riented organizations and academic institutions involved in
nternational activities. Often their expenditures on
foreign aid,: if calculated as "percent of Gross National
roduct" are greater than those of the U.S. That is parti-
ularly true for countries which still have strong ties
ith the peoples of their former colonial empires, like
rance, the Netherlands, and Britain. The relatively small
candinavian countries, Norway and Sweden, have an unusually
trong commitment to foreign assistance, not only in relation
 financial support, but also to human service. You will
nd a disproportionate number of governmental and non-
overnmental programs, as well as involved individuals
om these two countries serving in developing countries and
 international organizations.

(BILATERAL) U.S. GOVERNMENT ORGANIZATIONS

Governmental organizations range from the Agency for International Development to the Department of HEW with numerous activities that are more or less under the rubric of the Office of International Health (which officially represents the United States on the World Health Assembly of WHO) and agencies within other U.S. government departments.

The Agency for International Development (AID) is responsible for all federally financed and/or administered projects for foreign development assistance. Established under the jurisdiction of the Department of State, this agency is the only one in the U.S. government with the mission to help other countries to solve their development problems, regardless of immediate benefit to the U.S. Being a government agency, however, it is inevitable that its activities are influenced by political considerations to varying degrees. Health related programs are an important component of the multidisciplinary development activities of this agency. Their programs are frequently executed through contracts with private firms, other government agencies, academic institutions and individuals.

The Department of Health, Education and Welfare (HEW) maintains an Office of International Health, headed by an Assistant Surgeon General to direct and coordinate the international health related activities of the many components of this vast agency. Included under this rubric is the Fogarty International Center in the National Institutes of Health (NIH), as well as the many international activities offices in the individual institutes, such as the Geographic Medicine Branch in the Institute of Allergy and Infectious Diseases, and the National Library of Medicine. The Center for Disease Control (CDC), another agency of HEW, is in addition to its activities in the U.S., heavily involved in international programs. The worldwide eradication of smallpox for example was accomplished by a joint CDC-WHO campaign.

ser Departments, for instance, Agriculture, Army, Navy,
d Air Force have international health related programs
pending on their missions and interest.

derally chartered institutions such as the National Science
undation and the Institute of Medicine of the National
ademy of Sciences in addition to and in pursuit of their
tional goals, are paying attention to international problems.

ese governmental agencies and programs are only examples
the many international activities in the health field.
th the widely accepted broader definition of "health"
d the recognized multidisciplinary character of programs
med at improving health, the number of individual
ograms within the government is likely to increase.

N-GOVERNMENTAL ORGANIZATIONS

ny different private organizations are engaged in inter-
tional health programs, working sometimes in collaboration
th government agencies and often supported by them. Often,
ough, they have to rely on private financing. There are
re than 120 registered voluntary organizations with a
mulative international expenditure of funds that has
ipled in the fifteen year period between 1960 and 1974.
ring this period there also has been a shift in the
ographic targets for funds away from Europe and toward
ia, Latin America and Africa. Programmatically, this
ift has been accompanied by a change in emphasis from
manitarian relief programs (such as the CARE food packages
 war-torn Europe) to programs emphasizing planning,
aining, and evaluation in the health sector. Included
ong the non-governmental organizations are both non-
ofit and profit-oriented agencies.

ssionary and non-profit voluntary organizations are
e oldest (pioneer) groups engaged in bringing health care
d modern medicine to the developing world.

Almost all churches and denominations are or have been
engaged in varying degrees in this international
humanitarian effort. As a motivating force, missions such
as the one of Albert Schweitzer in Gabon, are unparalleled,
even though today rising nationalism and emphasis on local
solutions have created increasing problems for missionary
health work.

Other non-profit, humanitarian voluntary organizations have
become the highly effective successors to missionary work.
One example is Project HOPE, which operates in many developing
countries through local clinics and hospitals (after
abandoning the "Ship Hope"), programs of health worker
training and technical aid. Both missionary and non-
missionary humanitarian programs must be counted in the
thousands and their contribution cannot be overestimated.

Traditionally, foundations have supported international
programs and activities, not only financially, but also
through the participation of staff to help implement projects
in foreign countries. Often, these organizations are able
to use resources more effectively than government agencies
because they are immune to political pressures at home and
abroad and because their organizational structure lends itself
to carrying out programs without suffering the stigma of a
profit motive. A highly successful campaign against yellow
fever, for example, must be attributed to the resources and
structural make-up of the Rockefeller Foundation. (Examples
could be cited from more than fifty foundations engaged in
international health activities).

All international activities in the health field actually or
potentially can be of importance and benefit to the U.S. not
only from the humanitarian and economic/political points of

ew, but also in terms of academic knowledge and training. me universities capitalize on this opportunity by under- king international activities which enable them to amine different social and cultural phenomenon and explore e feasibility of transferring technical developments and ills to the conditions of different societies. A "general provement in the quality of life" being one of the aditional concerns of universities, the cooperation of thropologists, sociologists, designers, engineers, onomists and health professionals in defining the nature "development" beyond the too-narrow context of economic velopment is an important academic project. More than me of the other organizations involved in international alth, universities are independent of economic and litical considerations.

recent decades, particularly with the emergence of the l-rich developing countries, <u>commercial</u> <u>consultant</u> <u>groups</u> ve entered the health field. They frequently work under ntract with U.S. government agencies or with foreign vernments. In many instances these firms have shown markable organization and their performance record is ually excellent. On the other hand, it must be recognized at the need to please and agree with the customer can ad to an uncritical acceptance of the customer's wishes.

ULTILATERAL) INTERNATIONAL ORGANIZATIONS

lthough the health components of <u>SEATO</u>* and <u>NATO</u>** might looked upon as multilateral programs, the best example a multilateral agency is the <u>World Health Organization</u> HO).

Southeast Asia Treaty Organization
*North Atlantic Treaty Organization

The World Health Organization (W.H.O.) was constituted only after World War II, officially in 1948, as a single universal health organization. Previously, only partially accepted multinational agreements on international health methods existed, such as the Paris based "Office International de Hygiene Publique (O.I.H.P.) and the "Pan American Sanitary Bureau" (P.A.S.B.) for the Western Hemisphere.

W.H.O. is strongly decentralized. The six regions (see Figure 2) on page 13, each with a Regional Office and a Regional Director, are largely autonomous.

W.H.O., which has its Headquarters in Geneva, now forms part of what is commonly called the United Nations (U.N.) system. However, it is not a subordinate of the U.N., but rather "a specialized agency" attached to the UN by formal agreement. WHO has its own governing body consisting of the 140 member countries' General Assemblys and its own budget. While most countries are members of both the U.N. and of W.H.O., some countries (e.g. Switzerland) are only members of W.H.O. The funding of W.H.O. comes from contributions by the individual member countries, which all have the same vote even though the greatest contribution from the U.S. covers more than one quarter and the smallest less than 1/1,000 of the budget.

The fact that W.H.O. not only depends on the contributions of the individual members, but is also governed by the vote of all members, poses a problem for its activities. It is an international, not a supra-national organization, and often policy decisions are more influenced by political than by technical considerations.*

---

*For further discussion of the impact of political structure on health activities, see Unit IV/5, "Political Forces."

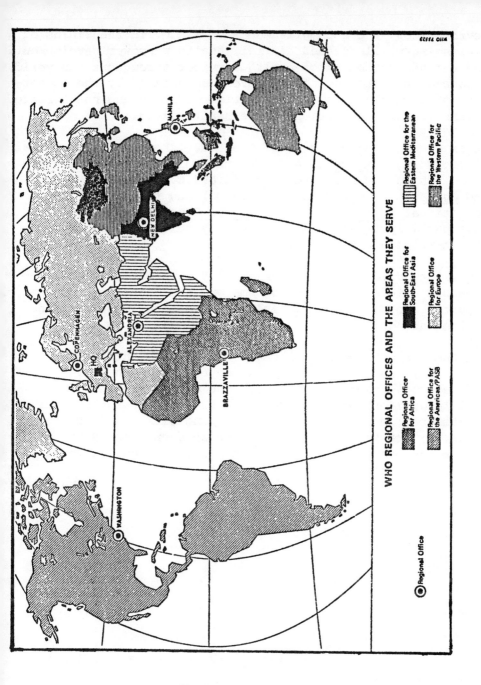

WHO REGIONAL OFFICES AND THE AREAS THEY SERVE

◉ Regional Office

▨ Regional Office for Africa

▨ Regional Office for the Americas/PASB

■ Regional Office for South-East Asia

░ Regional Office for Europe

▥ Regional Office for the Eastern Mediterranean

▨ Regional Office for the Western Pacific

WHO 73333

I/5, p. 13

Nevertheless, the accomplishments of W.H.O. in the fields of disease surveillance and control, health manpower development, and the strengthening of health services throughout the world, have been remarkable. It has promoted decisively the acceptance of public health and preventive medicine and has fostered international cooperation in the health field.

Other specialized agencies of the U.N. like the International Atomic Energy Agency (I.A.E.A.), the United Nations International Childrens Emergency Fund (U.N.I.C.E.F.), the Food and Agriculture Organization (F.A.O.) and the United Nations Educational, Scientific and Cultural Organization (U.N.E.S.C.O have participated with W.H.O. in many multidisciplinary health-related activities.

Also, the World Bank has increasingly gone beyond the simple financing of development programs and has contributed technica expertise to most multidisciplinary projects, which include health-care delivery.

All these organizations, because of insufficient funding and personnel, must rely heavily on cooperation with private and national government groups. The main strength of a multilateral organization rests in the universal character of its programs. Especially for coping with problems such as highly transmissable diseases which cannot be contained within the boundaries of a single country, a multilateral organization can be highly effective.

Quick Review

r each of the features on the left that relate to the
rengths and/or weaknesses of organizational types in inter-
tional health, select the <u>one</u> <u>or</u> <u>more</u> organizational types
om the right to which, in your opinion, the feature applies.
ep in mind that there are no objectively correct answers.

FEATURE	ORGANIZATION

_____1. Is subject to influence
by political considera-
tions

A. U.S. Agency for
International
Development

_____2. Motivated by humanitarian
effort

B. missionary and non-
profit organization

_____3. Has an official mission to
help other countries re-
gardless of the immediate
benefit

C. foundation

D. universities

_____4. Has a high performance
record but tends to be
uncritical of the "custo-
mer's" wishes

E. profit-oriented
consultant firm

F. multilateral agency
such as the World
Health Organization

_____5. Is best able to implement
programs that cross national
boundaries

_____6. Its international involve-
ment may be independent of
either economic or political
consideration

_____7. Its structure is relatively
immune to political pressures at
home or abroad.

WHAT ABOUT YOUR INTEREST IN INTERNATIONAL HEALTH?

Opportunities for international health work, not only for students but also for graduates and faculty members of health professional schools, are becoming increasingly more difficult to find. There are several reasons for this: in the developing world training institutions and programs have multiplied and often the need for expatriate, less trained and only temporary help has correspondingly decreased. Also, a worldwide increase in nationalism, and unfortunately sometimes anti-Yankeeism, has caused a reluctance to accept Americans. Financial support from various sources in the U.S. has also markedly diminished. All this applies particularly to unskilled or semi-skilled individuals, who want to remain overseas only for a short period of time and who expect to be paid.

Individuals with a special skill, for instance laboratory technicians, nurses, health care providers at all levels and basic science teachers, who are willing to spend as much as an academic year in one of the mushrooming health care delivery systems or training centers, including the many new medical schools, in the developing world, are still welcome, often even receiving a modest salary, or at least room and board.

Since there is no national or even regional organization in the U.S., which collects and distributes informationon these opportunities, you must almost entirely rely on the

lationships which your institution, your professional
ciety, your friends, and you yourself have developed.
me information and advice might be obtained from the
erican Medical Students Association (A.M.S.A.), the newly
rmed International Section of the American Public Health
sociation (A.P.H.A), the World Council of Churches in
neva, Switzerland, and interested faculty members in some
dical schools. A book on "U.S. Non-Profit Organizations
Development Assistance Abroad" (see References) can give
u some indication of opportunities and another book,
nnual Register of Grant Support" (see References) on
ssible financial support.

rtainly, planning for work overseas will require perseverance
d ingenuity. You should be prepared to be frustrated,
cause opportunities for untrained individuals and health
ofessionals in training have very markedly decreased in
e past few years. Naturally, full or partial funding by
ur institution, your family, or other personal sources,
ens many doors. If you can afford it, you should certainly
nsider paying your own way, particularly if you are in an
arly stage of your health career and therefore cannot yet
ntribute a great deal to the developing society.

owledge of the language of the country where you want to
rk is almost always a prerequisite. Also, an understanding
the cultural and social conditions of the host country
fore you arrive there, as well as knowledge of the health
oblems and the proposed solutions, is necessary to avoid
ur disappointment with the living and working conditions
u find yourself in, and your host's disappointment with
ur attitude and performance.

u also must be aware that wherever you go, you will find
eat curiosity about the American way of life, politics,
alth conditions and care, and you should be prepared to talk
out them, sometimes even in lectures and in conferences.
great deal of restraint is required to avoid being too

boastful about our standard of living and critical about the conditions of the host country. While in many instances and situations you may be acting as an "agent of change," this role has to be played very tactfully. All in all you must maintain a positive attitude towards your host country and towards your international experience.

WHAT ARE SOME OF THE MAJOR OBSTACLES TO INTERNATIONAL COOPERATION IN HEALTH?

Among the many problems, four particularly acute ones should be cited:

1. POLITICAL ENCROACHMENT INTO HEALTH CONCERNS

Both the increasing use or abuse by the donor nations of international health-related activities for political means and the rapidly mounting nationalism throughout the world have dangerously diminished the effectiveness and universality of international cooperation in this field. Even the U.N. affiliated international agencies have not been able to exclude political hostility from their activities and decision-making processes, which should be dictated solely by technical and humanitarian considerations. A strengthening of the supra-national rather than the international characteristics of these technical agencies would go a long way to avoid the danger of their politization.

2. MIGRATION OF HEALTH WORKERS

The migration of health workers from developing to the affluent countries is a serious cause for concern and friction. In a recent study by WHO (see reference), as many as 6% of the world's physicians in 1971 were practicing outside their own countries. Essentially, the affluent countries exert a "pull factor" by offering better living and working conditions and the developing countries add to this the "push factor" by training the physicians for

ctivities which their economic resources cannot support. As
s done already in many developing countries, an effort should
e made to offer such improved opportunities in order to retain
his manpower which is vital for further development. At the
ame time, affluent countries should see to it that their own
eaching and training programs are capable of providing their
ealth care systems with the required number of professionals,
hereby   eliminating the "vacuum" which attracts foreign
raduates at all levels.

ORGANIZATIONAL COMPETITION AND OVERLAP

ne of the principal problems lies in the large number of
rivate and government organizations which operate
ndependently of each other, and are engaged in often over-
apping and competing programs. The numerous bilateral
rrangements between national government agencies, private
rganizations, universities, and individuals, often without
verall planning and coordination, leave certain population
roups oversupplied, while others are underprivileged and
nderserved, though sometimes over-surveyed, because they
ffer "interesting" health conditions. Greater reliance
n the international organizations, particularly W.H.O., for
lanning and coordination in multilateral activities would
elp to remedy this problem.

ECONOMIC SHORTAGES

ne critical shortage of operating funds for international
nd national organizations concerned with health programs
as increased due to worldwide economic problems. With
nsufficient short-range funding for operations, funding
f teaching and training programs in international health,
n obvious long-range priority is even less available.
niversities, foundations and governments together must find
 solution to this vital problem.

UNIT REVIEW

This unit has attempted to explore the how's, why's and wherefores of international cooperation in health. Earlier you were asked to consider these questions and here is your opportunity to provide some answers.

1. Why do organizations undertake international health activities?

2. Name three types of organizations involved in international health and give a particular strength or weakness of each.

   (a)

   (b)

   (c)

Appraise the opportunities that presently exist for a career in international health.

Cite two obstacles to international cooperation in health.

(a)

(b)

*While the questions we have posed allow room for a variety of
subjective responses, perhaps you answered along the lines
of the following:*

1. Organizations may be motivated by altruism, a desire to
enhance political and economic stability throughout the world
by helping to offset the ever-widening gap between rich and
poor nations, and an interest in both sharing and learning
about new advances in health care technology and the organization of services.

2. (You could have named) in any order: (a) a _bilateral
government agency_ such as USAID, the HEW Office of
International Health or one of the other departmental
agencies of the federal government involved in international
health. (STRENGTH: Represents official position of U.S.
government; WEAKNESS: Is subject to political considerations).
(b) a _bilateral nongovernmental agency_ such as a missionary
or non-profit voluntary organization (STRENGTH: Humanitarian
motives); a foundation (STRENGTH: Immunity to political
pressure; structural organization conducive to implementing
programs); a university (STRENGTH: Its interest can be
independent of economic or political considerations); or a
profit-oriented consultant firm (STRENGTH: Geared for
excellent performance record; WEAKNESS: Geared toward
uncritical acceptance of "customer's" wishes); (c) a _multi
lateral organization_ such as the World Health Organization
(STRENGTH: Lends itself to the universal implementation of
health programs across national borders; WEAKNESS: Is
subject to the political pressures exerted by each member
state).

3. Career opportunities for U.S. citizens in international
health are presently waning because of (a) an increase in
the number of training institutions and trained health
personnel in developing countries, (b) a worldwide increase

nationalism, (c) a diminished proportion of global health
support presently being given by U.S. organizations, and (d)
reluctance to accept Americans, stemming from anti-Yankeeism.

You could have indicated two of any of the following:

(a) Political overtones whereas health matters used to
be apolitical concerns,

(b) the international migration of health manpower,

(c) inter-organizational competition and overlap, and

(d) economic shortages.

Some of the ideas presented in this unit you may wish to
discuss with your instructor and colleagues. For greater
depth, please consult some of the references which
immediately follow.

REFERENCES

Brockington, F. World Health, Churchill Livingstone, Edinburgh, London and New York, 1975
> An overview of the principal world health problems, with special elaboration of the history of international cooperation and the activities and problems of WHO.

Cahill, K.M., The Untapped Resource, Orbis Books, New York, 1971
> This book poses the challenge to the U.S. to use its wealth and power to fight ill health throughout the world. The author believes that this is "an untapped resource of contemporary international diplomacy."

Annual Register of Grant Support, Marquis Academic Media, Chicago, 1975-76
> A listing by subject, source, geographic area of grant and fellowships support in the U.S., including health related programs overseas.

Internationalizing the U.S. Professional School, Occasional Report No. 9, Education and World Affairs, New York, 1969.
> A collection of papers and conferences on "The Professional School and World Affairs."

Introducing WHO, World Health Organization, 1976

"Health Manpower Development. Progress Report on the Multinational Study of the International Migration of Physicians and Nurses," EB57121 Add. I, World Health Organization, Geneva (20 November, 1975).
> Report to the WHO Executive Board of findings describing an increase in the migration of physicians and nurses, particularly from developing countries to developed market-economy countries.

anpower for the World's Health, edited by H. v.Z. Hyde, ssociation of American Medical Colleges, Evanston, 1966.
   Report of the "Institute on International Medical
   Education" attended by numerous health manpower
   experts from many countries.

ar on Hunger, A report from the Agency for International evelopment, Vol. X, No. 7, p. 3.
   A bicentennial issue devoted to the role of voluntarism
   in the international health field.

orld Eco-Crisis, Edited by D.A. Kay and E. Skolnikoff, niversity of Wisconsin Press, Madison, 1972.
   A broad range collection of articles on successes of
   and constraints to international programs dealing
   with the environmental problems.

.S. Non-Profit Organizations in Development Assistance Abroad, dited by B. Crosby and S. Smyth, Technical Assistance nformation, Clearing House, New York, 1974.